Miracle Pill

10 TRUTHS TO HEALTHY, THIN, & SEXY

EAT THE FOOD YOU WANT

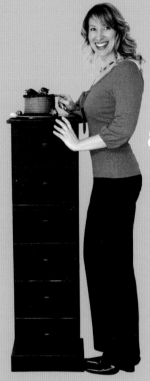

& STAY TRIM FOREVER

Tres Prier Hatch

TresBon Publishing

Alpine, Utah

www.miraclepilltruths.com

This book is presented as a reference volume only, not as a medical manual. The contents herein should help you make prudent decisions about your body and are not intended as a substitute for the counsel or advice of a doctor. Before beginning any weight loss program, please consult a competent medical professional.

All mention of specific companies, products, services, organizations, or authorities in this book does not imply endorsement by the author or publisher, nor does mention of such entities imply that they endorse this book. Any such recommendations or referrals are based purely on the opinion of the author. No money has been paid or received for these inclusions.

All references to specific trademarks, organizations, or resources were accurate at the time of publication.

Cover and book design by Daniel Ruesch Design
Cover Photographs by: Lindsay Jane Photography © Tres Prier Hatch
Other Graphics Courtesy of:
© Utah Department of Health: Adult Target Heart-rate Chart
© 2005 GardenShare Inc.: Eating with the Seasons in the North Country

ISBN: 978-0-578-04165-0

Printed in the United States of America.

Library of Congress Pre-assigned Control Number: 2009940193

TresBon Publishing
Alpine, Utah
tres@tresbonpublishing.com
www.miraclepilltruths.com

To Jon—
my best friend,
sweetheart,
father-of-my-children,
and shade of my heart.

Acknowledgements

First and foremost, I would like to say thanks to Jon, my husband. Your belief in this project has never waivered and your tireless patience with me has given me the strength and inspiration to go back to the computer, even when it seemed too daunting. You have put this work above "real jobs", which is unbelievably cool. I love you forever.

My three amazing kids—Kelsey, David, and Thomas—a huge hug and a kiss for your love and patience when I could not talk because I was trying to finish a sentence. You are my inspiration and joy. You are the reason I internalized these truths and took action. Please clean your rooms.

My parents, Peter and Kay Prier—the greatest cheering section this team ever had. Your witty and wise anecdotes dot the pages of this book because all that is best in me I learned from you. Thank you for contributing to this project: your love, prayers, patience, inspiration, and money, and for listening to me drone on year after year about the phantom book. It's alive....

John and Rene—my other parents, I cannot thank you enough for your tireless support of me, and our family. Thank you Rene for not only inspiring this book during our walks together, but also for providing me with your wise perspective on the topic. Thank you for your willingness to share your private thoughts and experiences with me, not to mention your beautiful photographs. You are hot, hot, hot! Dad, I love being your foodie friend. Thank you for the countless meals and recipes—you are a most unselfish man along with being the greatest baker I know, which is the highest compliment I can give.

My sisters Kris and Tammy—I cannot begin to thank you enough for putting up with my anxieties and pedantic droning. To have my sisters as friends means I never feel alone. Thank you for keeping me sane and reminding me to laugh at life, oh, and for feeding me. Kris—the cookies, oh yes the cookies. Tam—the cheese, oh yes, the cheese.

My brothers Marty, Paul, and Dan—thank you for supporting me through all the permutations of life. You taught me the kitchen table is a place for laughter—which is pretty healthy indeed.

Grandma—I love you. Thank you for a lifetime of unselfish acts and laughs. You are the hippest, most savvy, and most generous woman I have ever known.

My sincere thanks goes out to my line editor and friend, Heather Fry. You gave your precious time and talents even before we were close friends, or, as I used to marvel—for no good reason at all. Thank you for your generosity. Your edits were invaluable and helped shape this book while teaching me to cut "that."

One of the many answers to my prayers came in the form of my brilliant editor, Buffy Nelson. With each chapter I grew more amazed at your insight and wisdom. Thanks for sharing these gifts with me and for wading through my drivel of redundancy at a time when you were already nauseated. Your encouraging happy faces in the margins gave me the confidence to push on. Thank you.

Dan Ruesch—It has been a joy working together. Your brilliant design shaped a boring manuscript into something far more meaningful. I hope to work on many more hunger-inducing projects with you. Thank you.

An enormous thanks to the world's greatest General Practitioner, Peter V. Sundwall M.D. I might have stuffed the whole manuscript in a hole and buried it if not for your enthusiastic thumbs up. Thank you for reading it and immediately catching the vision. Your gracious quotes and comments in print and on camera were generous. Thank you a million times for your endorsements—I'm in your debt.

Dr. Richard R. Orlandi—you are pretty dang generous to your friends. Thanks for your willingness to take on my project, for your valuable time, and for your essential edits. Most of all, thank you for your quote and for your willingness to be a part of this book—it means the world to me.

Dr. Brandon Allen: you really owed me nothing, yet you said "yes." Thank you for spending your valuable time looking over this book, your edits, and for the encouragement.

My beautiful friend Laurie Olson can do anything—the proof is in the script and film direction for the book preview video—which you gave to me as a gift! There just aren't words for how much I admire you. You did an amazing job on this and all the projects we have laughed and cried over. Thank you for teaching me about patience and kindness in the home. I shake my head when I think of all the support of this book you have offered. Love you beautiful.

Aimy Kersey—no one sponge cakes or Bakewell tarts like you. Your support and encouragement are the loveliest gift I could ever imagine. Despite the ups and downs we have both experienced, you make life fun and inspire me to keep my chin up. Thanks for listening to my anxiety-ridden diatribes on life, family, children, money, and food, but most especially, thank you for your friendship and love. I cannot wait to tour French markets. Save me some cheese…

(Elder) Ollie Kersey, you prodigy—thank you for sharing such awesome talents with me. You squeezed in my no-account project at a time when you had better things to do, and it turned out fantastic.

Paul—thanks for lending Ollie out, for your generous business advice, the countless happy hours in your home, your outside-the-box thinking, and your friendship. I owe you all a tremendous debt.

Christian Olson, no one teleprompts or eats salad on-camera like you. Thank you for your easy generosity with me. I adore you.

Thank you to my friend Jeanne Engberson, who has taught me what I want to be when I grow up. Those early presentations to your T.O.P.S. group were really the catalyst for this book. Without your delightful encouragement, this project might never have made it to the page. Thank you for your friendship and for the bazillion acts of kindness you have shown me that I did not deserve. Stuffed cabbage is dedicated to you.

Tammy, your granola is essential to my day. You are my hero. Melanie Fitts, your cookies are medicinal. Michelle Sundwall, your easy crock-pot chicken is divine and kind of fits my schedule. Aimy, fantastic tarts! Marguerite Henderson, you guided me with a shared passion for food—the scone recipe is largely due to my excellent experience in your kitchen. Joe and Christy, your dumplings have been on the top-ten request list since the first bite. Chrystelle Francom, can I just clone you?

Maria, how can I repay all your efforts on my behalf? Helping me get connected with promotion in the Northwest, your ceaseless interest in this project, hosting many visits to the chez Wald spa and resort, your general belief that I am funny—all are just small parts of the priceless sisterhood we share. I love ya babe. Mark—thank you for your immediate friendship and trust. I am honored to be your wild game consultant.

Colette, thanks for the cake—which is really the tip of the frosting iceberg of your many impressive gifts. Thanks for your friendship, which I treasure.

I have been blessed with the many supportive friends including: Alise, Ruth, Sue, Katya, Klara, Crystal, Katie, Kay, Jacob, Michael, and dozens of others—you know who you are. Thank you for being true sisters and brothers, and for delicately nudging me to get the book out: *"Hey, stop lollygagging and finish the book already!"*

Marjie McCloy, you taught me much about writing. Thank you for all the kindnesses and opportunities you have given me.

Can I just proclaim greatness for my spectacular legal consultant, Adam Ford, of Ford and Huff. I marvel at your very big brain. Thanks for the landmine aversion counsel. Shaleen, I am in awe with your ability to smile through the "stuff" every day. Thanks for being a light in this world.

My thanks for the generosity of the Utah Department of Health's Heather Borsky and Barbara Larsen, for allowing the use of their Beats per Minute Chart.

My gratitude goes to Phil Harnden at Gardenshare.org, for the Eating With the Seasons Calendar. Your graphic conveys the information far better than words alone.

Stephanie Francom, I marvel at your ability to progress. I want to hold onto your ankles and end up where you are going. Thank you for inspiring the "rule of halves." You make life look pretty good.

My wholehearted thanks goes to Jaleh Fiddler for her expert skills as a "reader." Your first impressions were hugely helpful in providing me the confidence boost to get it done.

Awesome April Moriarty—your fireside presentation made a HUGE impact in my life and my husband's. Sometimes service ends up touching that "one person" and in our case, that beautiful night of violin music and inspirational talks was clearly just for us. Thank you.

My friend Stephanie Pinegar—your scanner saved me on more than one occasion. For the many times you said "yes" when a normal person would tell me to "get lost," thank you.

Ann Orton, you always made me feel special and your willingness to refer me to colleagues helped inspire a smidge of confidence just when I needed it. Plus, the cupcakes were to die for!

Debbie Simmons at Deseret Book—thank you for taking my calls, for trying to connect me with the muckity mucks, and for sounding interested over the phone. Not all new authors receive such kindness.

To all those who requested a copy in advance and to those who contributed recipes either directly or indirectly, I feel touched by your support. I hope it meets with your approval.

Finally, to my Heavenly Father and my Savior Jesus Christ, to whom I owe it all—to offer my love is spectacularly insufficient, yet true. The insights on these pages were inspired by Him—because all good things come from God.

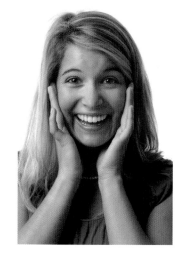

1

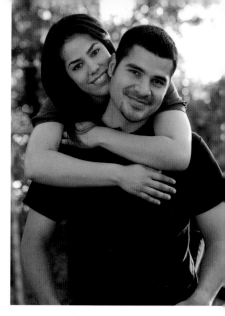

5

Contents

33

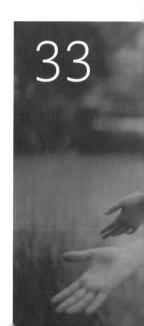

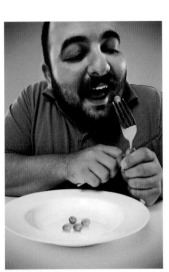

17

51

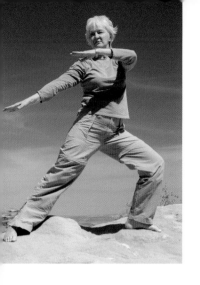

63

The 7th Truth: Consistency Not Intensity 77

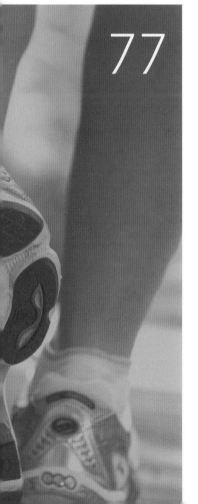

77

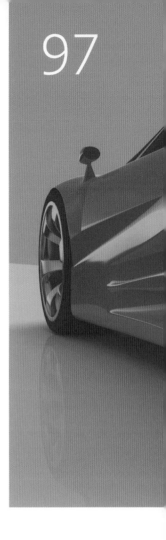

97

109

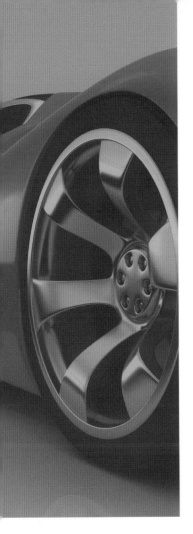

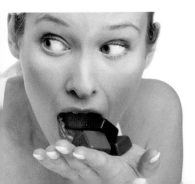

131

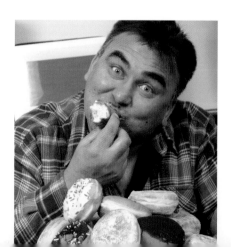

Miracle Pill *10 Truths*

1. Get the click

2. Health is beauty

3. Diets make me fat

4. Change the inside and the outside will eventually respond

5. What I think, say, and do, I become

6. Does my health program pass the test: …'til I'm 80?

7. Consistency not intensity

8. Treat my body like a Ferrari™

9. Quality, not quantity

10. Choose fuel my body wants, not what my mouth wants

Preface
·············

I am taking the liberty of making three suggestions on how to best use this book:

1 Please subject this book to hard use. Read with a pen and mark it up; make notes in the margins; treat it as a working manual. *Miracle Pill* is not intended to be another dust-gathering self-help book sitting unused on the shelf. When your personal notes and food splatters dot the pages and the binding is worn, you will have your money's worth.

2 After reading each chapter, give yourself time to think on the concepts you've just read. Try to apply each *Truth* to your daily life before moving on. Live each *Truth* one at a time, building on behaviors you already learned. Marinate in the ideas and play with the new paradigms. Experiment. See what works with your schedule and tastes. At the very least, give yourself time to absorb the material so you can change the way you think.

3 Many of the *Truths* in these pages were gained while I was praying on my knees. My Heavenly Father wants me to be happy and it is through His inspiration I learned these *Truths*. I received them because I asked, and because they are essential to my physical journey. There are many paths to the same destination and my solutions may not be the only ones. You can receive personal counsel regarding your body. Extend an invitation to the Lord to teach you through prayer. Just be humble, have faith, and ask. He knows exactly what you need to gain loving respect for your body. He knows because he made you and you are His child. All you need to do is ask in faith.

Disclaimer Because people tend to sue each other, I need to include the following disclaimer: I am not a medical doctor. This is not a medical book. Nothing I have written in this book should be considered medical advice. This book does contain general health and wellness suggestions but is not intended to replace the care of competent medical professionals. Please consult your doctor before beginning any weight-loss activities. Talk to a trusted health care advisor about how to incorporate into your life the general principles found herein. Individual results may vary because we all are different.

Please use wisdom to prevent injury. Any activity that can harm you or cause strain should be avoided.

Introduction

The funny thing about weight loss is it's not about what you eat or how much you exercise: it's about how you think. Our thoughts dictate our actions. In order to have energy, health, and lean muscle tone, we must think like a person with energy, health, and lean muscle tone.

In order to change the way we think, we must first be willing to give up the habits and comforts that block our desired outcome. Everyone wants a trim body. But not everyone is willing to let go of the *desire* to eat a dozen doughnuts. I am not talking about resisting the urge; I am talking about actually relinquishing and replacing the desire to eat an excessive amount of doughnuts or anything else for that matter. Imagine your results if all your impulses were the ones that would make you trim and vital.

This book is designed to do what no other health-management program purports to do: it changes the way you think. *Miracle Pill* presents a new way of looking at yourself and your behaviors. If you want weight loss but also want to hang on to your *desire* for a dozen doughnuts, you will have no better luck with this book than any other health-building program. However, if you are willing to submit to changing your desires, your impulses, and triggers, you can become a new person and your body will assume a different shape. So, if you have hit proverbial "fat rock bottom" and you want to change the way you think, read on.

The main body of this book is roughly grouped into three sections, with each chapter devoted to one

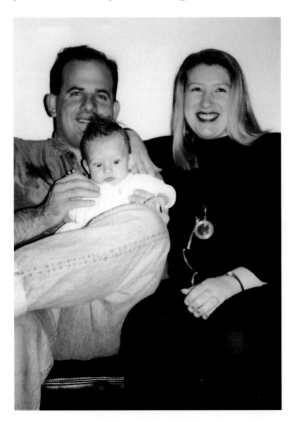

Here I am at 235 pounds (beginning to learn the 10 Truths). Seated beside me are my husband, Jon, and our new baby.

Truth. The first section is comprised of the first four *Truths* (chapters 1-4), and focuses on common-sense concepts you may already know and, hopefully, validates them as wisdom. The second section (chapters 5-7) should encourage and motivate you to look inside yourself and help you view exercise in a new way. The third section (chapters 8-10) deals specifically with how to choose the right fuel for your body. Throughout the chapters are 21 Tips designed to help you overcome roadblocks in your pursuit of health. In the reference section at the end of the book you will find a troubleshooting dialogue along with sample menus of a typical, balanced day. Because great food is a salient part of a healthy lifestyle, I also included dozens of recipes at the back (these are tested recipes of real food, not diet food, to help you eat abundantly), along with pantry stock recommendations.

Your time is precious, so the following *5 Touchstones of Successful Weight Management* are the five most powerful actions I would suggest. These *Touchstones* will help you quickly shift your thoughts to an enlightened place. Use them daily and refer to the back of this book for cutouts of these and other motivational thoughts.

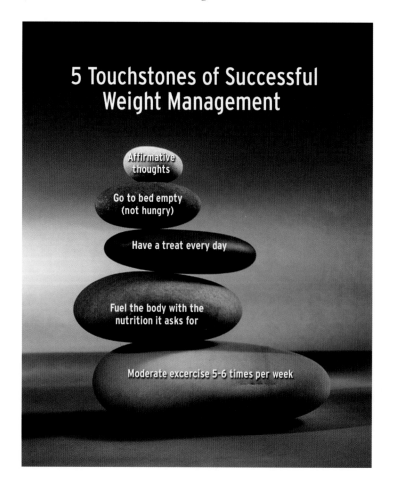

5 Touchstones of Successful Weight Management

Affirmative thoughts

Go to bed empty (not hungry)

Have a treat every day

Fuel the body with the nutrition it asks for

Moderate excercise 5-6 times per week

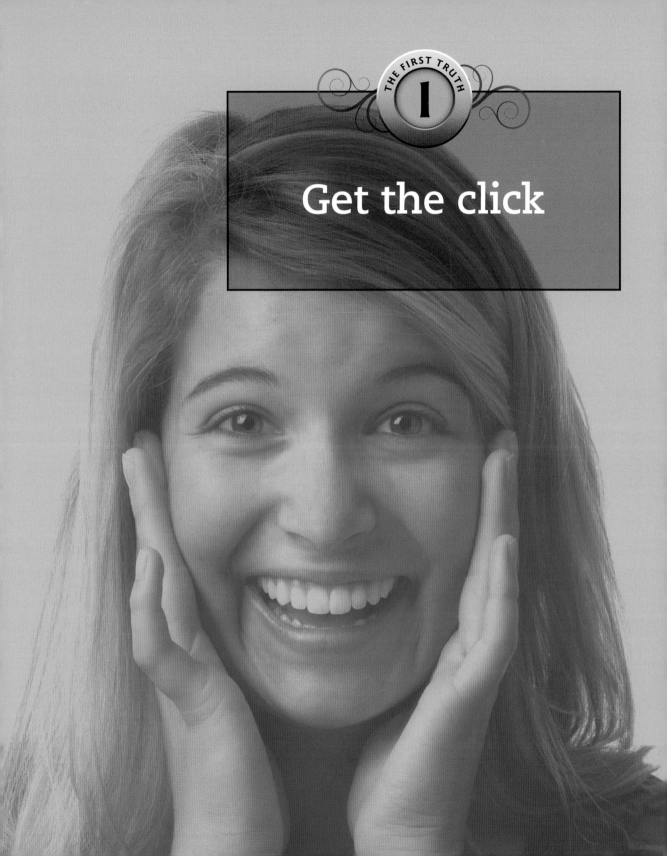

Get the click

Over fifteen years ago in a hospital bathroom, I stared at my naked body in a mirror and did not recognize the woman who looked back at me. I had just given birth to my first child following a very difficult pregnancy and my reflection was a grotesquely bloated caricature of the girl contained within. I was obese to the degree that I could not see myself behind all that blubber. I wanted to rationalize the weight away by blaming the pregnancy. After all, didn't every woman look fat right after delivering a baby? But, the baby weighed only 7-pounds, so how could I explain the extra 90-pounds still hanging on me? Even by post-pregnancy standards, I was extremely overweight. The truth was, whether the weight was gained from pregnancy or from aliens injecting me with fat while I slept, losing 90 pounds was a pretty overwhelming mountain to climb. And boy, oh boy, did I feel overwhelmed. I gulped and considered my options.

On the one hand, I could do what I had always done, which was of course, to diet. All my life I had been the "big-boned" girl, fervently searching for the ultimate program that would make me into a thin person. I had tried every diet on the market and even invented ones of my own. I tried the no-carb, the all-carb, Slim-fast®, low-calorie, low-fat, Weight Watchers®, Jenny Craig®, NutraSystem®, multiple juice diets, Cambridge®, The Grapefruit Diet®, Herbalife®, vegetarianism, aloe cleanses, and lots more. I exercised intensely on and off, suffered through years of anorexia, bulimia, depression, and even ended up in the hospital from overdosing on diet pills. My body and I had clearly never agreed on a weight management system.

This first option didn't seem very promising.

Option number two, on the other hand, was really the golden egg of weight loss: to somehow become a different person—a healthy, thin person. But, becoming a different person entirely was like grasping some elusive mirage in the desert. Living healthy was not an experience I could draw from. I knew people who had done it, but I wasn't exactly sure how I was going to do it. I very clearly saw two roads ahead of me. The road I was most familiar with always ended in the same place—dieting and then gaining the same weight over and over. But now, with a daughter to take care of, I could no longer risk my health and endure all the craziness as I had in the past. I needed to travel down a new road.

It was at that moment I had a very spiritual experience. Despite the unattractive flesh in the mirror, I felt God's love for me. I saw my body as a truly remarkable gift, warts and all. From my Heavenly Father's perspective there was only love for me and for my rotund body, and a wave of acceptance washed over me. In my mind came the distinct thought, *"There is a beautiful girl inside this body, even if I cannot see her right now. But God can see her and He thinks I am beautiful....I better not argue with God."*

It was as if there was a *click,* like a switch turning on in my mind, and it shored up my courage to become healthy from that moment on.

My first order of business was to stop the invective tirade in my head. I realized that within my private thoughts I constantly criticized myself. I thought horrible things like, *"You are so disgusting, you fat pig!"*

And the first few days after I left the hospital, I caught myself thinking these things every few minutes. It took effort to preemptively catch the punishing thoughts enough to stem them. After about a week I noticed I had quelled the nasty word-storm for a whole day. Imagine how good I felt that day. I went around whistling with a bounce in my step. The sheer weight of that much self-abuse was an enormous burden to carry around and I was not even aware I was doing it until I stopped.

More wisdom followed and over time new paradigms became habits—which basically means I changed the way I thought and behaved. The following chapters reveal each in detail. Because I was actively seeking answers regarding the management of my body, I did not take lightly new *Truths* as they presented themselves. The profundity of each *Truth* became quickly apparent. Unlike a fleeting thought or random idea, these 10 *Truths* distilled in my head and heart so intensely as to be incorporated not only on an intellectual level, but also felt on a physical level. My body actually proved them to be, well…true. As my thoughts changed, my behaviors began to change. Eventually, my body manifested those changes by shedding excess fat. Amazingly, I learned how to eat what I wanted and not be fat.

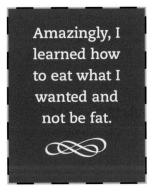

Amazingly, I learned how to eat what I wanted and not be fat.

The concepts in this book apply whether you need to lose 10 pounds, 90 pounds (like me), or 290 pounds.

Have a Moment

It all started with a "click." With humility and an open mind, experience your own profound moment. If my story resonates with you enough to stir a desire for change, you are right now experiencing a "click" and I urge you to keep reading in order to learn new patterns of thought. Maybe you have already felt a deep stirring to become a different person. Perhaps your turning point is yet to come. Moments of significance come when we are teachable. When that moment comes, don't ignore it or chalk it up to wishful thinking—act on it. Without action, those progress opportunities don't propel you anywhere and they become wasted.

My husband had a teachable moment while reading an early manuscript of this book. After trying for several months the principles taught herein, he realized his lifelong pattern of intense exercise for a week or two followed by the absence of any exercise for months formed an ineffective and frustrating baseline. The "click" for him was realizing his baseline could be moderate "easy" exercise on a regular basis—5-6 times per week. Walking and slow jogging was much more effective at keeping his weight in balance than whip-lashing back a forth between "too much" and "nothing." He now keeps trim with a sustainable habit and when life throws a recreational basketball game or snowmobiling into his day, he feels fit enough to enjoy it and then go right back to his baseline of light exercise the next day.

Find your click and believe permanent change is possible.

* * *

Miracle Pill is simply a tongue-in-cheek term for giving my body great fuel and exercising consistently. That's it, no magic secret. And, unless you have lived in a cave for the last 30-years, you already know eating well and exercising are *the* formula for fitness. This is not news to anyone. The real challenge is changing our behaviors in a permanent way, seeing the world through a new lens, anchored in a desire to eat healthy and exercise regularly. Shifting from being one kind of person to a permanently healthy person is the real "miracle" in *Miracle Pill*.

So, as a result of taking this *Miracle Pill*, I am more beautiful. I am smarter and will likely live longer. I am healthier with fewer aches and pains. I have more energy. I am happier, sexier, and more confident. The bottom line: my bottom line will never be fat again.

By internalizing these *Miracle Pill* concepts, I have learned to enjoy food again, to really taste and stop worrying about my weight. I take pleasure in eating, without any guilt. Additionally, I look forward to active movement. I am now in control of my body for the first time in my life. I will never again follow a diet program of any kind. No more calorie charts, meal plans, counting fat grams or carbohydrates, avoiding sugars, or shelling out lots of money to follow someone else's structured plan. I've said goodbye to weight fluctuations. The holidays now come and go and are marked by how much I enjoyed my loved ones, not by how many pounds I gained between Thanksgiving and New Years.

This book is the antithesis of the belief that "thin-is-everything." It challenges the notion that health is secondary to beauty. It presents a different model from the "denial" mantra that permeates our diet-obsessed culture. We were designed by God to enjoy food and take pleasure in eating. It would be unwise to pit my strength against the will of The Creator by denying myself pleasure. Therefore, the question remains—how do we reconcile two seemingly opposing objectives: fulfillment at the table while maintaining a healthy body?

I will answer that question in the following pages, but just to complicate things further, in my own life I work with food as a TV chef, caterer, food writer, and food educator. I am up to my elbows in great eats all the time and I like it this way. I live to eat. Because food is very important to me, I simply will not settle for less than delicious food—without compromise. So how does a "foodie" become balanced, thin, healthy, AND satisfied forever? The answer is *Miracle Pill*.

Here is the next ingredient:

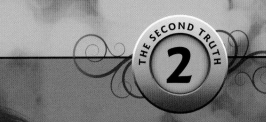

Health is Beauty

Because, if you don't have your health, you don't have anything...

THE PRINCESS BRIDE

We all want to be good looking. Let's just admit it. We go around espousing the merits of great cardiovascular health and squeaky clean intestinal tracks, but when we get down to it, we all want to look gorgeous on the outside. We want to be attractive and wear clothing sizes in the single digits.

When I was an obstinate teenager, my Mom used to say, *"Dear, health is beauty."* Meanwhile I would exercise three hours straight and eat M&M's™ and Diet Coke™ for breakfast. I did not believe her. I was convinced skinny was beauty. Just look at any TV show, magazine cover, or movie poster. Thin (not healthy) is the common thread that runs through all those pretty images. It took me twenty more years before I started understanding what Mom meant.

To completely make the point that "health is beauty," I urge you to consider celebrities who are not aging gracefully. We have all seen famous people live hard and become prematurely old and bloated. Sure, a nip and a tuck will freshen them up, but that only makes them look unnaturally weird. Sadly, plastic surgery does not last and Father Time catches up with them with a vengeance.

Without a balanced lifestyle, unhealthy behaviors eventually become visible on the outside. Unhealthy is ugly. Even the prettiest face in the world looks haggard when it is hanging in the toilet with the stomach flu. Case-in-point: *health is beauty!* Thin is not the ultimate prize. Health is the *Miracle Pill*, and trim is the happy by-product of healthy.

I once saw a documentary on the fashion industry. Prior to a fashion show, all the models arrived without makeup, fancy hairstyles, lighting, or costumes. They were sickly, gaunt, and tired with cigarettes hanging out of their mouths. Some threw back a drink or two just to get in the mood to sashay down the runway on those tiny little legs. Some snorted cocaine. Watching this, all I wanted to do was feed those poor starving girls. Not one of them was beautiful. They all looked precarious

> **Thin is not the ultimate prize. Health is the *Miracle Pill*, and trim is the happy by-product of healthy.**

as if one gulp of smog would finish them off. It wasn't until they were all gussied up that they looked good enough to be sent out in designer clothing—and even then, they looked in need of a hot bath and a free bowl of soup.

It was reported that during the golden age of Hollywood, the famous makeup artist, Max Factor, was asked which studio starlet had the best figure. According to legend, he replied "Greta Garbo, for about five minutes." In other words, in real life, even movie stars cannot maintain the level of perfection we expect from them for more than short stints of time. And the media chronicles their fall from grace with gleeful zeal. Apparently, we eye-candy, celebrity-obsessed sycophants want something from our stars other than what can be achieved with good health and a balanced life. The price is too high if it demands extreme starvation and excessive methods. Why, then, should we demand it of ourselves?

Think of someone you know who has a balanced life and takes great care of themselves. Whether that person is the Swedish grandmother who walks her dog every day or the fifteen-year old captain of the soccer team, their forms reflect strength and balance; their eyes shine and their skin glows. Think of the people you know who are healthy from the inside. These people are beautiful, and will keep their beauty.

* * *

If health is beauty, let's explore health.

In simple truth, good health means having enough energy to fill our lives with the things we want to do: catch a Frisbee™, hoist a tire, chase a toddler. Good health includes the ability to sleep regularly, respond to our bodies when we are hungry, drink when we are thirsty, and eliminate wastes comfortably. It means our systems and organs function optimally and our minds are clear and effective. In short, a healthy person feels well enough to work, play, and handle the ups and downs of life.

Sure, there are lots of solutions to gaining "health." You can spend a fortune on things that are supposed to make you healthy. Adding a new supplement to your diet or a new exercise to your routine at the gym may be healthy activities, but they are only part of the formula for overall health. Don't get seduced into marketing campaigns that promise if you buy *their one thing*, it is going to make you healthy. A total lifestyle of healthy behaviors practiced in moderation over the course of time brings about health. Sorry, there are no shortcuts to health-ville.

So, what is the foundation of health?

Balance is Health

A healthy body is a balanced body. Balance is the key. Even on a cellular level, our bodies have a delicate balance of things flowing in and flowing out; such as water and electrolytes passing in and out of cell walls, creating balance at all times.

In order for our skin to look even and smooth, our skin cells must constantly slough off old dead cells, exposing new skin beneath and achieving balance between the old skin and the new. Our respiratory system is another obvious example of our body's need to be balanced. We inspire air into our lungs and then exhale waste gasses (carbon dioxide among others). In and out from the moment we are born until the day we die our bodies maintain equilibrium and balance.

The circulatory system is a marvel at keeping a balance between nutrient-rich blood and nutrient-deficient blood. In fact, all body operations require a perfect balance in order to serve us well. When that balance is interrupted, it puts a strain on our body systems. They don't work as well, we do not feel as well, and we don't have as much energy. We are more at risk of illness and injury. Our bodies emit bad odors. (And, I don't care how beautiful you are, gassy is not pretty.) Due to imbalance, we age at a more rapid rate and then we die. Imbalance is not very exciting to say the least.

Of all we do to affect our health, maintaining balance in these three areas has greater impact on our overall well being than anything else:

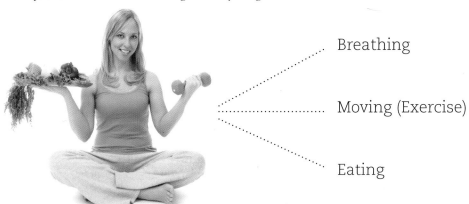

Breathing

Moving (Exercise)

Eating

We breathe in and out all day long, we move constantly, and we eat at least three times a day. Considering the regularity of these things, it is no surprise they are going to make or break our goal to fit into sexy jeans. If one or more of these things are not in perfect balance we certainly feel (and look) the imbalance.

Let's examine how much impact these three things have on our health.

Breathing (Oxygenation)

"The utilization of fat always requires oxygen....The amount of oxygen available to body cells affects the proportions of fat and carbohydrate that will be used for energy production." (J.L. Christian and J.L. Greger, 105)

In order to increase metabolic rates and burn excess fat, we must maintain a balance of sufficient oxygen. But, you ask, don't we get enough oxygen from reflexive breathing in and out? If you tend to gain weight during periods of inactivity, the answer is no. It is during physical exertion that we increase the saturation of body systems with oxygen-rich blood—thus speeding up our ability to metabolize fat.

Normal talking seems like a good way to increase oxygenation. However, to speak the English language, minimal air is required compared with other languages. As a nation of "shallow breathers," our speech patterns do not demand rigorous exhalations. When tethered with inactivity, the end result is we do not take in enough oxygen to efficiently metabolize our food. To counter this, deep breathing every day will encourage our metabolisms to burn fat for fuel—and nothing makes us breathe deeply like exercise. Team up deep breathing with exercise, and we create a fat-burning machine.

"But I move around all day long in my job!" Why doesn't normal daily movement provide sufficient oxygen to our bodies? In our urban world, we don't move much as part of our daily activities. When was the last time you had to carry water from the well? Or bale hay? Or dig furrows in the dirt? Or hike a mountain to flush out a bird to shoot for dinner? We shuttle our bodies around in cars. Don't get me wrong—I enjoy my washing machine as much as the next housewife. The increased comforts of modern technology *have* extended the average life expectancy in developed countries by almost double that of 200 years ago. This is a good thing. But, compared with our ancestors, our lives are sedentary. For the last 20,000 years, the human body has succeeded with a tremendous amount of physical activity. Exercise increases respiration. Without enough activity, we don't breathe deeply enough and our brains, muscles, and organs become oxygen deficient. It is a marvel we can count fat grams on a box of cookies with as little oxygen as we have going to our noggins.

The good news is we can make up the oxygen deficit with a moderate amount of daily exercise. It doesn't take anything too extreme. Regular cardiovascular exercise elevates our respiration to a rate that feeds our body with oxygen. This in turn speeds up our metabolism. Ideally, we should spend time both sitting at a desk and moving our fannies. As a caution, please don't decide to oxygenate by gasping for air or you'll just hyperventilate and fall down the stairs. Instead, try the following breathing technique adapted from yoga visualization practices. Balance is the goal.

Breathing Technique

Make a point to inhale and exhale deeply a few times each day and, for maximum benefit, during the peak of your daily exercise. To get started, inhale through the nose with mouth closed, and exhale out from the mouth. Picture oxygen as colored vapor entering the nose and circulating throughout your body. Imagine the air traveling from the tips of your fingers to the tips of your toes. On an exhale, picture the vapor leaving your body. With each inhale and exhale, fill every inch of your body with energy and healing.

A more advanced technique involves breathing audibly through both the mouth and nose, opening up the throat to make a rasping noise. This is most effective right in the middle of your workout. Hold the breath in at the top of the breath and then exhale, pausing for a beat before talking the next inhale. Continue with the "vapor" visualization for an energizing, relaxing pick-me-up.

It is highly effective to combine breathing exercises with cardiovascular exercise. However, you will benefit any time from oxygenating your body. Try breathing in the car or while working at a desk. When people are around you might need to use the quieter technique. Try it right now. Picture the colored air circulating in and out. It feels good and elevates the mood. Read more about the benefits of oxygen at the end of Chapter 7.

Exercise

Any discussion about exercise and its role in balancing the body should start with a short list of some of its cleansing benefits.

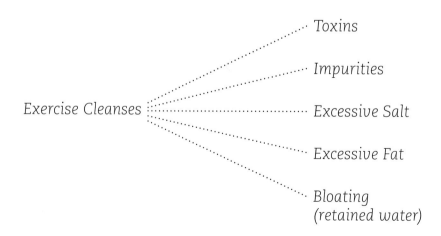

Exercise Cleanses

- Toxins
- Impurities
- Excessive Salt
- Excessive Fat
- Bloating (retained water)

I once asked a physician to estimate what percentage of ailments could be prevented or successfully treated with regular, moderate exercise. A wide range of health problems were included in our discussion, including hypertension, diabetes, cancer, knee problems, and everything in between. This physician honestly felt eighty percent of the "typical" physical challenges that plague us would be eliminated with consistent exercise. Either they would be prevented entirely or they could be minimized by the benefits of exercise. Eighty percent! It makes sense when we understand that all systems of the body are connected. In order to maintain balance in one part of the body, the other parts must be fed with proper nutrients as well, and exercise is the great equalizer. It restores our cells to an optimal state by providing them nourishment and eliminating waste. It compensates for the slice of chocolate cake I ate last night. It makes me sleep better so I have better recovery from moving my furniture this afternoon. It keeps me flexible and active. It helps stimulate my bowels in the morning. And, it reduces anxiety.

Exercise Reduces Anxiety

With our demanding lives it is no surprise we have more anxiety disorders than there are names for. Prescriptions written for anti-anxiety medications are at an all-time high. Stress-reducing services like massage, yoga, and meditation studios are part of the fastest-growing industry in our country. Clearly, we need healthy techniques to decompress and stabilize our minds and bodies on a daily basis. Exercise is a highly effective de-stressing technique because it allows our own body chemistry to go to battle for us. As we stress, we secrete toxins into our tissues. As we exercise, our endorphins absorb and eliminate these toxins, leaving us cleansed of fatigue-causing agents and our immune systems boosted.

While exercise is standard therapy for adult patients with anxiety disorder, you might find it interesting that a classic treatment for anxiety in children is joint compression. Parents of clinically anxious children are taught to gently compress the child's joints starting with the wrists and moving up to the elbows, shoulders, ankles, and knees. Parents are also encouraged to have the child jump up and down to compress the joints. A trampoline is ideal for this exercise. Joint compression effectively reduces stress and anxiety in the toughest of clinical cases. Imagine the benefits in the general population of regular jogging, dancing, walking, skipping rope, or weight training. As you do the low-impact version of these activities, you compress all the joints in the body and receive anxiety relief. Read more about exercise in chapters 7-8.

Eating—the Impact of Food

We eat three times a day (at least) and yet we seem to underemphasize the correlation between health and what we eat. We ask our doctors for pills, supplements, and surgical procedures to fix what could be prevented with correct nutrition. Not all conditions can be remedied with nutrition after the fact, so the cure really is in prevention. Few things make a greater impact on our overall physical well being than eating, because we do it multiple times every day.

After twenty years of forcing too much of the wrong fuel into our gullets, it is no wonder excess fat shows up on our thighs, and our ankles start to hurt from the added burden.

Even too much of a good thing will put a strain on the body. We have become a

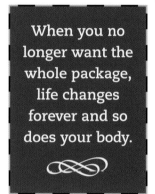

When you no longer want the whole package, life changes forever and so does your body.

nation of fat people eating entire packages of "fat-free" cookies because we are under the misguided notion they are "good" for us. There is nothing wrong with fat-free cookies, but when I polish off the box in one sitting because I consider it a "freebie," I am clearly not listening to my body anymore. There are too many carbohydrates, refined sugars, and salt in a package for me to eat more than one or two cookies. It is our *desire* to eat the whole package that this book addresses because when you no longer want the whole package, life changes forever and so does your body. Keep reading to learn how to eliminate cravings that are out of balance with the fuel you require.

Why do I want the whole package?

Well, arguably, because it tastes really good. But, perhaps there is more to it. Why have we deactivated that "done" mechanism we had as child that told us to stop after one bowl of ice cream? (See *Full Mechanism* in Chapter 3, for more specifics about how this works.) In the meantime, let's answer the question: Why the whole package?

One reason we eat excessive amounts is because we stop tasting the food. You can protest and swear you tasted every last one of those Fritos™, but I challenge that. Overeating is usually distracted eating. Whether we are stressed, bored, or self-punishing, when we eat more than we need (often referred to as a binge), our souls go elsewhere. Rather than living in the moment and savoring each bite of pie, we transport our minds somewhere else, using food as a vehicle of escape. The more we binge eat, the less we feel satisfied because we have not tuned in and tasted. Add to this dynamic the accompanying guilt we feel afterwards and what do you get? The bingeing cycle: An unfulfilled desire to escape, coupled with great imbalance in our bodies and a side order of self-loathing. Chapter 8 deals more with the trap of bingeing, but the following graphic illustrates this classic bingeing cycle.

THE BINGEING CYCLE

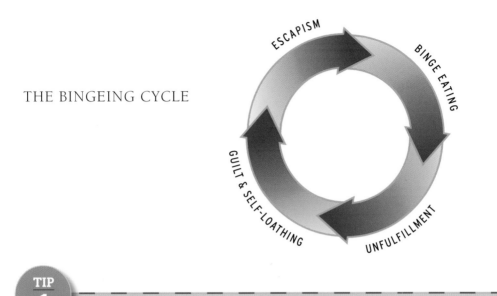

TIP 1

Savor Food Concentrate on tasting your food. Really savor it.

In our society there is a lot of guilt loaded into every fattening food. We think, *"Yikes, potato chips and onion dip. I can't. It is just too good. I won't be able to stop. I shouldn't…well, ok, maybe one. But, I won't think about it while I eat it because then the guilt will set in…I'll just chew while my mind wanders off…"* When was the last time you enthusiastically enjoyed butter?

Because we idealize "skinny," we have onerous clouds of food guilt hanging over our heads. When we acknowledge the deliciousness of food, it is no wonder we escape to another realm and don't taste. We eat, but heaven-forbid we taste. What self-respecting person would eat fattening food with their head, and fork, held high?

This book presents an alternate point of view. Why not tune in and taste? Enjoy every bite and you will be satisfied with the amount that your body needs. No guilt. This is the attitude of a thin person, a lifelong healthy person. Go ahead, eat that cheese omelet with buttered toast, savoring each bite for all its worth. As long as you let your body dictate when you eat and how much, you will stay thin while enjoying great food. Keep reading to learn more specifics.

A Tasting Exercise

Don't settle for mediocre food or else the following exercise will be useless.

1   Choose the best quality food you can afford—not necessarily gourmet but fresh and well prepared—and eat some. Tune in to the taste, texture, and temperature. Analyze the flavor profile, determining levels of sweet, savory, salty, bitter, etc.

2   Decide if you actually like the tastes and textures of your test food. During this process of discovery, you may decide you don't like those store-bought tomatoes, and only home-grown tomatoes on the vine really appeal to you. Shortbread cookies made with real butter might reveal themselves as heavenly compared to the blah taste of those commercially made. You may feel far more satisfied enjoying only three bites of a great brownie than you would from a whole package of cheap, store-bought, processed, overly-sweet, loaded with shortening, flavorless garbage. High quality food tastes better, something that is revealed immediately during this exercise.

3   Log these preferences away for future reference. Every time you eat, choose what you truly like—not just what is there. Hold out for the good stuff.

4   Do this exercise every time you eat, even when you are snacking on something small.

5   If you find the texture or taste unappealing, stop or spit it out. However, if you find the taste heavenly, sit quietly in the moment and enjoy it. Never feel guilty for enjoying fantastic food. After eating consider carefully if you want more or if you feel satisfied (if you have had enough). Recognize the moment when eating something sweet or rich goes from being delicious to unappealing. Pay attention and respond when you get a prompt from your brain saying you are "finished." When you really tune in, that prompt will come. Your portion size will shrink as you practice this exercise of focused tasting because less food will satisfy. Remember, eating for pleasure is healthy, using food as an escape is harmful. See Chapter 8 for more on this.

The amount and the quality of food we eat *most regularly* determines how we look and feel. When looking at amounts, remember, unless you are training for the Iron-Man™ triathlon, the typical restaurant portion size is twice what you need for optimal balance. Most people don't scoop a mere ½-cup portion of ice cream into a bowl. Yet, that is a reasonable portion size if you do not want to store that ice cream around your middle.

In terms of the quality of food we regularly eat, junk food may not exactly be poison, but it has little nutritive value. And, you'll have to work very hard to use up all those calories unless you want to store excessive fat on, let's say, your upper arms. This is not to say you should never again eat a Twinkie™, it just means whatever your normal diet consists of will shape your weight, energy and overall heath, good or bad. If Twinkies™ are part of a normal day, you, my friend, are going to wear the effects.

When your choices consistently reflect a desire for quality fuel at the right time and in the correct portion (balance), your body takes on the optimal size and shape. Health really is beauty. The following chapters identify ways to shift our desires so they are in sync with our needs. You heard right—our desires can be changed. Remember, this book is not a diet book. It helps you change your mind, and when you change your thinking, your actions automatically adjust—and so does your pant size.

Miracle Pill focuses on how to reconcile our two national pastimes:

1 How to eat the delicious food we want

2 How to remain slim and healthy

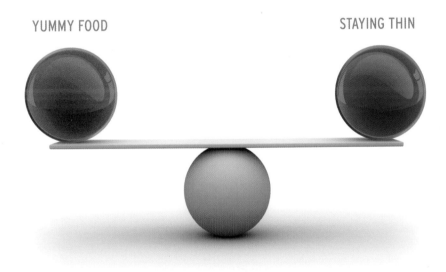

YUMMY FOOD   STAYING THIN

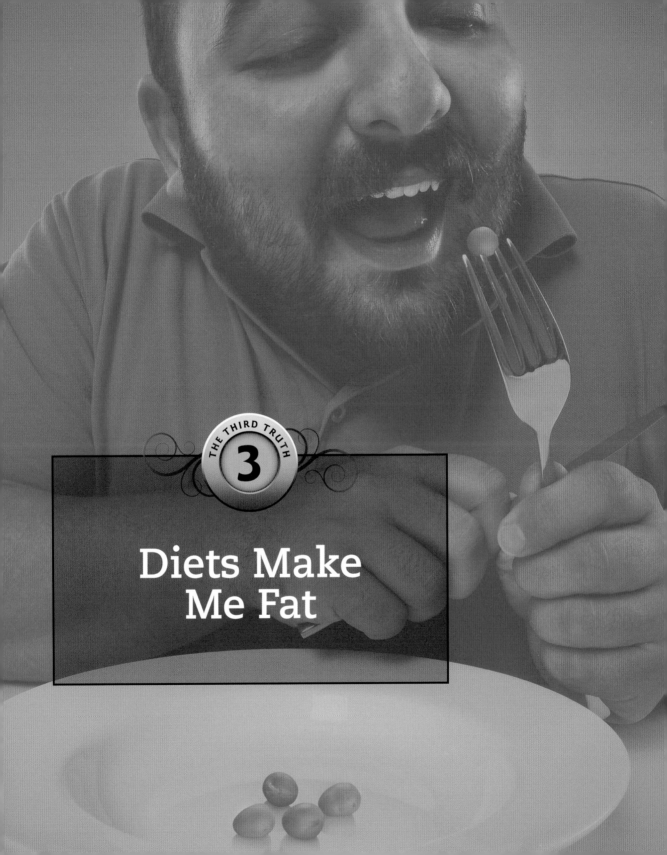

Diets Make Me Fat

The Wrong Promise

Diets sell you the pitch of weight loss. That's all. They don't promise you will overcome fat issues. They only suggest you might temporarily lose weight, and even then you have no guarantee—*"Individual results may vary."* Think about it. When was the last time a diet promised you it would make you a healthy, trim person for the rest of your life *without continuing their program?* They are in business to make money and would like very much for you to be their best customer, but make no mistake, they do not promise permanent freedom from fat issues—because only a healthy lifestyle can do that. Sure you may lose weight on a diet, but that elusive goal of becoming *both trim and healthy* is not the end result of most programs. They even admit their program does not produce lifelong health. Included in the directions in fine print are instructions how to wean you off their program—called the "transition" or "maintenance" phase. Implicit is their admission that their program is not the solution to lifelong health. However, the maintenance phase—the part you do all by yourself—*is.* But they will happily take your money until you figure it out.

Many of us, including me, are gullible consumers: *"If I can just lose the weight, I will worry about the maintenance later."* Sound familiar? The fantasy of *thin* is so beguiling, and we are so desperate, we don't care if maintaining that weight loss is virtually impossible. We want to be thin *if only for a day.* The weight loss industry is acutely aware of these feelings among their target demographic.

Another deception is the promise that their product makes it easy to lose weight. They make it sound like you are only along for the ride while they do all the weight-loss work. The truth is: only *you* can do the weight loss part just as only *you* can do the maintenance part. Save your money and start with the maintenance phase or, as I like to call it, healthy living.

> **Marketing campaigns promise to do for us that which we can only do for ourselves.**
>
> ⚮

Learn to cultivate the habits of a healthy person, the kind of person who stays trim and active their whole life.

We are a society of people who have learned to distrust our body's signals and buy into clever advertising. Marketing pitches promise their product or program will do for us *that which we can only do for ourselves.* Programs and products are not the answer. Your success will be the result of a paradigm shift from trusting products with a big marketing budget to trusting yourself, believing your body, and listening to the prompts it makes. Relying on your own common sense more than the "quick fix" offered by strangers who want your money. Your body has the ability to direct you to what it needs, as you have probably discovered from the *Tasting Exercise* in Chapter 2.

How Did I Become This Way?

To fully make the argument "Diets Make Me Fat," I must first be truthful in answering the question: How I did become this way? Let's look at the following formula:

Behaviors—acquired or learned

Metabolism—genetics

+ *Wild cards—illness/injury/pregnancy/medications*
_____

The State of My Body Today

My behaviors, plus my metabolism (which is largely genetic), plus wild cards over which I have no control, combine together to produce the state of my body today. Let's break them down individually to determine what I do and don't have control over.

Behaviors—habits

Some behaviors are acquired, others are learned, but regardless of how they came to be part of my world, I still have complete control over my behaviors. I might abdicate that control to a litany of bad habits, but, in truth, they are still bad habits I can change. Chances are that a whole pizza and pint of ice cream weren't shot out of a cannon, landing unexpectedly in my mouth. You can bet I ate them of my own free will and choice—same thing with the now-empty bowl of M&M's™ by the television. I find it liberating to assume responsibility for my habits and recognize they are mine to change if I choose.

Metabolism—genetics

We each came to earth with our own unique metabolic rate. Someone with a fast metabolism has a hard time keeping weight on. Those with a slow metabolism tend to gain weight easily. Although our metabolism may be genetically programmed, our behaviors can speed it up or slow it down. For example, a 53-year old woman, who has been overweight her whole life and has never exercised regularly, can shift her metabolism into a fat-burning machine with consistent moderate exercise and better nutrition. Metabolic rates can increase. Even people born with enviably fast metabolisms find their bodies slow with age and they start gaining weight in places they never did before. This effect can also be countered with increased activity and better fuel for the body. In short, our behaviors can affect our metabolisms. Hence, we have *some* control over our metabolism (more on metabolisms later).

Wild Cards

There are some factors I don't create or have control over. Some "wild cards" include: menopause, side effects from medications, depression, childbirth, injury, etc. I don't get to choose the metabolic effect from these conditions. The good news is I can manage these situations with optimal behaviors to minimize the slowing of my metabolism and the creation of bad habits. Many concepts in this book can be generalized to address the specifics of your unique situation. But the point is: my behaviors are something I can change, and they also give me some control over any wild cards in my life.

Diets Don't Work Because...

Now that we have taken an honest look at how we became overweight, we can dispel the myth that diets are the solution to a weight problem.

Let's pretend we go on a diet and lose 20-pounds. We have now been off carbohydrates, sugar, fruit, meat, dairy, or too few calories in general—and we crave it. The restricted food now becomes our binge of choice. (You know how out-of-control we get when we take a day off from the diet. We go crazy and eat massive quantities of the forbidden food.) In addition to this binge response, the following three critical diet flaws identify fundamental reasons why diets are counter-productive to the goal of healthy lifelong weight management.

Critical Diet Flaw #1—We Have a Survival Mechanism

One problem with diets is that they make our metabolisms slow down and encourage our bodies to store fat. Our bodies are designed to protect us from starvation. When we do not have enough fuel, our metabolism slows down to a snail's pace, and instead of burning fat for fuel, it increases the likelihood we will store fat. Anyone who has gone on a diet and found they were gaining weight on 1,200 calories a-day can tell you this is a fact. If we put our bodies in starvation mode they will stave off the perceived famine by storing fat.

It is not only low-calorie diets that trigger this starvation mechanism. Any imbalance to our systems can create the same result. To keep our bodies burning fat and revving at full throttle, we must fuel them with high-grade food. Specifically, we need correct food at the correct time.

What happens if, due to a diet, we become saddled with a slow metabolism, and then we binge on the very foods we have been deprived of? You guessed it: we hop on the strudel express; in other words, we gain weight and we gain it fast. Usually, we gain back what we lost plus extra pounds. Our self-image goes down the disposal and we feel even more desperate than before. Calorie cutting and food restriction do not work.

Critical Diet Flaw #2—No Permanent Change

A major flaw in dieting is the fact that at no time during my diet have I done anything to permanently change the very behaviors that made me fat in the first place. By design, a diet is a temporary thing. It is like a vacation from my regular eating habits.

"Oh, but this time I am going to stick to it for the rest of my life," we promise ourselves. Who can live the rest of their natural life drinking a meal replacement shake twice a day? Going without bread, eating pre-packaged freeze-dried food, or any of the other crazy things we do that are now so commonplace in our society that they don't even seem crazy any more.

Diets not only lack the ability to teach healthier habits, but they can also program our bodies to crave unhealthy food. For instance, let's say we drink a powdered shake for two weeks. This does absolutely nothing to change my behaviors except, perhaps, to teach me to want a chocolate shake every day. So, when we go off the diet (*and we will because it is a temporary fix*), we simply return to the habits that originally made us fat plus we now have an unnatural desire for chocolate shakes.

$$
\frac{\textit{Slower metabolism} + \textit{Unhealthy behaviors}}{\textit{Weight gain}}
$$

Critical Diet Flaw #3—Ignore Body Prompts

Another major flaw is that diets inherently require us to tune out the needs of our body—forcing us to ignore our body's messages.

"I must be strong and ignore my craving for a piece of bread"

Here is something the fifty billion dollar per-year diet industry does not want you to know: Your body is designed to ask for *what* it needs and it will tell you *when* it needs it. A healthy person listens to the needs of their body. Today if you are very active your body may tell you to eat protein. Do you need more hydration? If so, you will feel like drinking more water. Need a treat for pleasure? Yes, even pleasure is a need and your body will tell you when it wants that too. The need for whole grain and exercise and seasonal fruits and vegetables… these are all messages your body will give you at exactly the right moment for your health.

How does this message-system work? Have you ever noticed a beautiful vegetable in a produce market and wanted to eat it? It just looked so good you could almost taste it right there? Or, have you ever craved the cool juices of a ripe peach or chilled watermelon on a hot summer day? Those impulses are telling you that you need the nutritional value and hydration of those foods. Translate those prompts into every meal choice and you become healthy. Listen to your body. It will send you healthy cravings as readily as unhealthy cravings.

> **Listen to your body. It will send you healthy cravings as readily as unhealthy cravings.**

Vitamins and minerals are frequently combined with weight loss products to make them sound more "healthy." Don't be fooled. Nutrition originates as food. We should get our primary nutrition from what we eat and not rely on supplements to make up for substandard fuel. We live in an age when every good food available on earth is found in our markets. If we need it, we can get it. Take advantage of the bounty of the earth to give your body the vitamins and minerals it asks for.

If you listen and give your body what it wants when it wants it, you will become balanced and your system will run at an ideal metabolic rate. However, if you follow a diet plan which makes all the choices for you, it is not likely to be compatible with what you need *that day*. Diet plans invariably exclude various food groups (like carbohydrates) from your day, which means you have to ignore the messages your body is sending you in order to stay on the diet. When you crave a potato, you probably need the wealth of B vitamins, antioxidants, and carbohydrates contained within this starchy root. Denying yourself a potato because it doesn't fit with your diet program may actually slow down your engine and inhibit weight loss. Sure, refusing the potato may mean you ingest fewer calories, but you won't train your metabolism to burn hotter by withholding the essential fuel it asks for. Giving your body what it needs is fundamental to speeding up your metabolism, creating balance, and establishing habits that lead to lifelong health. Remember, the goal is to be trim and healthy for the rest of your life, not just until your 20-year high-school reunion.

Start listening to the promptings of your body. If a salad sounds good but you are at a famous rib and barbeque restaurant, go for the salad. It will taste better than the ribs. Really, it will. Need proof? Have you ever been really thirsty? You know how wonderful a cool glass of water tastes when you are parched? Nothing tastes better than that water. The same principle applies for food. When you give yourself what you really *need*, it tastes fantastic. We will talk more about food choices in Chapters 8–10.

Drink Away the Munchies Sometimes we get the munchies. Maybe we are not exactly hungry, but we just feel like eating something. Most of the time, that craving is really thirst. Next time you feel like chomping some chips have a tall glass of water and wait ten minutes. You may find the craving is satisfied.

Full Mechanism

Another remarkable system our bodies come equipped with is our "full mechanism." This natural gauge tells us when we have had enough food. As we eat, our digestive system activates multiple hormones that deliver messages to the brain, telling us we are satisfied—to stop eating. Hormones such as DHEA, manufactured in the brain and adrenal cortex; HGH—human growth hormone, produced in the pituitary gland; CCK, from the intestine; and other hormones are responsible for a sated feeling. Unfortunately, many of us have deactivated this mechanism by ignoring it and overeating. Some people don't ever remember feeling full as a child and may need to activate this system for the first time in their lives.

If you don't believe there is such a mechanism watch children eat cake at a party. They dig in to a piece of cake, all gooey with frosting, and for a few precious minutes it is silent. Two-thirds of the way into the piece of cake, the children look up and push the cake away. Just like that they are done. They run off to play without another thought of the leftovers on their plate.

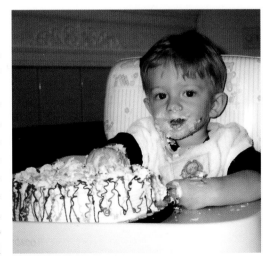

Everyone can reactivate their full mechanism. All you need to do is behave as if it were working. Try this experiment: after five minutes of eating, sit back. Enjoy some conversation. Give your body time to catch up with your stomach. If you decide to dig back in, don't feel obligated to finish everything on your plate. Stop before you feel full. Have some pleasant conversation. At this point imagine how you would feel if you got up from the table to do something active. If you feel energized and satisfied, you consumed the correct amount. If you feel swollen and lethargic, stop eating and make a mental note for next time. Choose to indulge in this experiment as frequently as you need, at least for the next few meals. After a few days or weeks, your hormones will start sending you full signals. You will eventually establish the habit of listening to the promptings of your body and recognizing your limits. Your full mechanism will re-activate.

Chemicals and Supplements

In order to become balanced, it is crucial to hear your body's directions. Therefore, avoid anything that overrides your ability to hear. Abstain from impulse-suppressing chemicals like caffeine, tobacco, alcohol, and most especially, diet pills.

Diet pills have only one purpose. That purpose is to mask your hunger promptings. Sure fat melts away—because these chemicals suppress your impulses to eat while your nervous system and blood pressure shoot through the roof. Not good. Remember what happens to our metabolism when we stop eating? Imagine the strain on your organs to be pumped full of unwanted drugs and then to go up and down in weight.

Universal laws dictate when you give nothing, you get nothing.

Diet pill manufacturers bank on our greed. They want us to think we can accomplish something great without doing anything except taking a tiny little pill. Universal laws dictate when you give nothing, you get nothing. In order to become healthy we must actively *do*—specifically engage in moderate daily exercise and eat great food.

Even scarier than pills are some of the new radical weight-loss programs that try to hook you with "easy" weight loss. The latest craze involves injecting fat-melting human growth hormones into your stomach and hips. Really? That is not right! Weird stuff is not sustainable forever and it is probably dangerous. Every couple of years we see lawsuits and massive recalls of powerful weight-loss drugs and schemes. These products jeopardize our health and put us at risk of things far worse than fat.

Meal replacements and powdered formulas are usually so full of sugar that an hour after eating them you cannot recognize whether you are really hungry again or just having a sugar low from the resulting insulin spike. With regular consumption, these products can wreak havoc on your metabolism, slowing it down and making you fat.

Even worse are products containing synthesized sweeteners and fats. These sugar and fat substitutes have been around for decades, but recent advancements have resulted in *seemingly* innocuous products flooding the market. Unless you have a medical condition (like diabetes) that requires sugar substitutes, please avoid fake food. Chemically engineered molecules are hard for your body to recognize and process correctly. Fat substitutes are particularly scary.

Your system does not know what to do with fat-altered molecules because they cannot "hook up" with other molecules naturally and therefore pass right through the system. Printed on the package of foods containing synthetic fat is a health warning claiming their product may cause digestion problems including "anal leakage." I don't know about you, but if I have to choose between anal leakage and being fat, I would rather be fat!

To all you diet soda drinkers: recent study findings officially dispel the myth that low-calorie diet soda will keep you thin. It won't. In fact, doctors now believe daily consumption of diet soda could contribute to excess weight.

Since the 1950's most artificial sweeteners and synthesized fats have faced government recalls and health warnings. The latest one just came under scrutiny this year. It doesn't take a medical degree to see the pattern and wisely avoid these ingredients. I refuse to put engineered fake sugar in my body.

Even health supplements can be problematic when it comes to tuning-in to your body. Many herbal supplements are in combination with "natural" stimulants that increase your blood pressure and make you sweat more. Some supplement formulas contain untested ingredients that essentially turn you into their guinea pig. Use good judgment when choosing any vitamin supplement. The notion you can eat all the low-grade fuel you want and just take a vitamin pill is untrue. Pills cannot replace the process of speeding up your metabolism with optimal fuel and regular exercise. Sorry, they just can't. Enjoy the wealth of nutrition found in food.

Having said that, there are valid medical reasons for taking supplements. Many people are unable, for one reason or another, to absorb or produce enough of a certain nutrient. For instance, smokers do not absorb vitamin C very well and may need to take it in supplement form. We also know aging bones benefit from a daily calcium supplement. So, construct your diet so a supplement is only a small piece of the overall puzzle and not a substitute for good old-fashioned healthy food.

I once had a conversation with a woman who was earning thousands of dollars every month selling vitamin supplements through a network marketing company. She extolled the virtues of her products and bounced on the balls of her feet with excitement as she shared her joy that she could make so much money doing it. Fishing for a new customer, she asked me how much I spent every month on supplements. When I informed her I don't take any, her jaw dropped. "You mean you don't take any supplements at all?" I told her I eat my vitamins—in my food. After thinking this over for a moment, she leaned in and conspiratorially whispered that with the money I saved each year on supplements I could probably take a trip to Hawaii.

Unless you have a valid medical need, eat great fuel and save your money for a vacation.

Another confirmation that I was "on track" came several years ago when I was scanned for nutritional deficiencies at a demonstration sponsored by a well-known skincare company.

Naturally, they were selling supplements they thought I was in desperate need of. Knowing my body was in good balance, I warned the sales representative not to use me as a test subject. Despite my protests, he insisted I take the scan in front of several other prospective customers. So, I placed my finger on a read-out pad and after a minute or so, the computer generated a number. Upon reading it, the company rep seemed perplexed by the results and immediately punched in a request for a second reading. Once again he stared at the results in disbelief. Because I was out of time, I prodded him to give me the results and he reluctantly handed me a certificate (see below). It indicated I was off-the-charts healthy and I

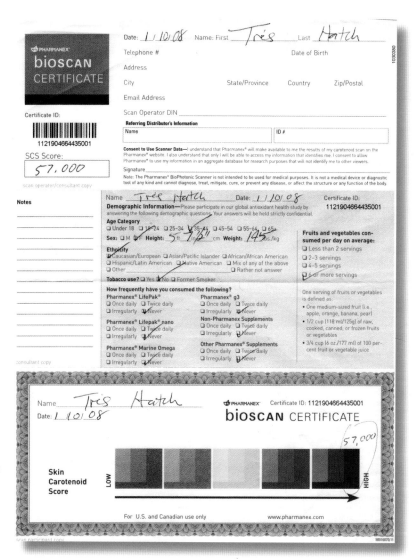

This certificate was given to me when I was scanned for nutritional deficiencies at a supplement demonstration by a Fortune 500 company.

had no deficiencies. He admitted most people, whether fat or thin, register a number between 12,000-30,000. My number was 57,000, defined by their own system as an extremely high saturation of nutrition. The others witnessing all this asked me what supplement product line I was taking and *could they buy it?*

Our need for nutrition through diverse, seasonal, and delicious food is a natural requirement of our programming. Of course, we don't need new technology in order to live healthy and strong. Every time I hear about a "revolutionary" product or program, I laugh. Extolling the benefits of simplicity, noted inventor and scientist, Ray Kurzweil, wrote in his book *The Singularity Is Near*, "*Simply having more information does not necessarily result in a better fit. Sometimes, a deeper order—a better fit to a purpose—is achieved through simplification rather than further increases in complexity.*"

Kurzweil then goes on to quote another famous thinker:

"Make everything as simple as possible, but no simpler." —Albert Einstein

Our bodies are designed to become healthy and strong with optimal fuel and regular moderate exercise—without the use of synthesized products. In fact, the more unprocessed (simple) and natural our fuel, the healthier we become.

Metabolism

Now, let's talk a little more about our metabolisms. Metabolism is the rate that our bodies use the food we consume and the fat we have stored. If balanced, our metabolism rapidly burns fat for fuel and uses sugars quickly. If you want to remain trim for life, it is important to encourage a fast metabolism. It can be your best friend or your worst enemy. You probably know exactly which way your metabolism is leaning right now. Even small behavior adjustments, over the course of a year, can result in metabolic acceleration. Diets, on the other hand, slow down a fast metabolism, as explained previously in the *3 Critical Diet Flaws*.

We all know someone who seemingly eats anything they want and never gains weight. I used to whine about the injustice of it all. Then I came to terms with the fact that I must manage my body without comparison to others. Who cares if cousin Bob can eat a whole pizza without gaining a pound? Bob's horking down pizza doesn't have anything to do with my body. I will exercise regularly and eat a moderate diet because that is what *my* body needs. Complaining about what other people eat, or how unfair is life, does not get me the results I am looking for.

How do you transform your metabolism so it works in your favor? The formula is:

Consistent Exercise + Quality Fuel Going In = ↑ *Metabolism*

That is it. You have heard all the noise about shortcuts to skinny-ville and I am just here to confirm that you were right all along—there are no quick fixes. Only healthy food and lots of moderate exercise will create a fat-burning body. Please don't get discouraged and go looking for an easier track. Read on to learn how to change your desires so you *want* to eat well and you *want* to exercise.

Exercise Increases Metabolism

Exercise affects the rate that we burn fat: Following a workout, our bodies continue to burn fat at a higher resting rate. Expending a set value of calories during a workout is not nearly as beneficial to weight-loss as is the metabolic boost experienced over the 24-hours following exercise. So, not only do our bodies burn fat for fuel during a workout, they will continue to use up fat stores the rest of the day and night, even while we sleep. Our bodies can become fat-burning machines and all we have to do is plug in daily exercise to make it work. If you hate to exercise, read Chapters 6-7 because they deal extensively with changing negative paradigms regarding exercise.

Portion Size

Another way to accelerate the metabolism is to reform portion sizes. Although portion size was briefly mentioned in chapter 2 in the section: *Why Do I Want the Whole Package?* this topic deserves more than just a cursory word or two. Sometimes we *want* a big bowl of cereal, but don't *need* a big bowl of cereal. Taking bigger portions than we need is more habit than anything else. To change our portion choices, shift thoughts away from "How much *can* I eat?" to "How much do I *need* to eat?" Say the second phrase out loud.

Thinking differently means portioning out food differently. It is a useful tool to portion out your food so you consistently have just enough or less than enough. If we finish a small portion and are still hungry, we can always take more. However, if we consistently take more than we need, we tend to consistently eat more than we need, because, like Mount Everest, it is there. So, start with the rule of halves explained in the next section. I learned this rule from my good friend Stephanie Francom, who dropped over 20 pounds while eating the foods she wanted.

The Rule of Halves

Try the rule of halves for two weeks until you see a noticeable difference in how you feel after a meal.

At each meal take about half the amount you would normally take. This is not to restrict your calorie intake, but to re-assess your correct portion size. Most of us eat more than we really need (don't worry, you can always take more). After eating your half-portion meal you should feel comfortable and satisfied, but still be able to suck in your gut. You should feel energized. If you need to unbutton your pants make a note to take even less at the next meal. Go for second helpings only if you *need* it. Initiate the tasting exercise from Chapter 2 because it slows down your eating and allows your brain to figure out if you have had enough or if you really need that second helping.

Be picky about what food groups you take seconds from. A meal comprised of one carrot stick and a bowl of noodles is not exactly balanced. It takes multiple vegetables and a myriad of colors to fulfill your nutritional requirements (see Chapters 9-10). If, after initially taking half-portions of chicken, salad, and rice, you are still hungry, take a little more of whatever your body needs. Listen. If it asks for more protein, choose more chicken. If you need more carbohydrates, dish up a little more rice. Does the crunch and hydration of salad sound good? Then help yourself to more greens and vegetables. Stop when you start to feel full—not when you already feel stuffed. With practice, you will become very efficient at gauging the exact quantity of food at each meal for your body. Over time you may notice weight loss. If you don't, please rest assured, reducing your portion size in concert with regular exercise will produce weight loss. It might take time, but it will come.

Beware of cutting back portion size for

Don't Be Afraid of Hunger.
Don't worry about feeling hungry when you cut back on your portion size. Hunger is an indicator that your metabolism is doing its job, processing fuel, and burning fat. That gnawing hungry feeling is a good thing. But, we don't want to experience hunger for more than an instant so when you feel hungry: eat. Every time you hear the message to eat, answer your body's request with food. Keep small, healthy snacks available to stave off hunger until mealtime or, if it is time for a meal, choose balanced foods your body wants. Handfuls of granola, berries, raw nuts, soybeans (edamame), fresh or dried fruit, sliced turkey or chicken, tuna fish, eggs, cut-up raw vegetables and dip, whole grain bread, string cheese, and other "whole foods" are great for taming the "flaming hungries." Avoid loading up at meals to prevent hunger. It is unlikely you will get lost in the desert between lunch and dinner. Just eat whenever you feel hungry.

the sake of cutting calories. You need enough fuel for your body to run at optimum speed. Too little food will cause you to go into deficit and mess up your metabolism. Too much food and you don't lose weight. Find the balance for your particular body.

"Fattening" Is a Dirty Word

Now that we have discussed quantity of food, let's talk about the cliché: fattening verses non-fattening. My dear friend asked me once if my granola recipe was fattening. I didn't know how to answer her question because *nothing is fattening.* Two bites of a brownie is not fattening when I want a small treat. A smear of cream cheese on my whole-wheat toast is not fattening if my body needs it. Decide what to eat by what you need, and by considering what you've already fueled your body with today. My granola happens to contain a lot of whole grains and some protein. If today I already had lots of grain (cereal, bread, etc.), then no granola for me, because I don't want to overwhelm my body with too many carbohydrates in one day. If I haven't, then I say yes to the granola. The granola is not fattening, it simply may not be part of a balanced day relative to what I have already eaten. Instead of counting carbs or calories I try to balance between the food groups, avoiding too much of any one group. Don't get hung up on the details. Think in generalities. For instance, if I had eggs and toast for breakfast I might choose vegetables and fruit for lunch. Simple.

Too often we label a food "non-fattening" only to consume it in greater quantities than we need, or we eat it when we don't need it. *Any food* taken in excessive portions or at the wrong time is not good for you. Lose the notion of good food and bad food. Focus more on listening to your body and balancing choices.

Throw out food restrictions. There is nothing wrong with mashed potatoes and gravy if your body wants them; keep in mind a healthy body will not want them every day. Enjoy them while observing the rule of halves. You may find after only a few bites your tastes are saturated with the rich gravy and starchy potatoes. Heed that cue and stop. Doing so will guarantee future prompts from your body. When you feel no restrictions, you will feel satisfied with the quantity your body directs you to eat.

TIP 3

Nothing Is Fattening Don't choose food based on whether or not it falls into a category of fattening or non-fattening. Make food choices based on what your body says it needs and what you have already had today.

The Two Blacklisted Foods

Out of the entire spectrum of edibles in the world there are two primary foods I simply try to avoid: hydrogenated fats (shortening), and high fructose corn syrup. They are both processed and altered in a way that makes my body store fat. Having said that, I am not going to pick out only the filling in my cherry pie, and leave the crust behind, just because Grandpa made a traditional pie crust with shortening. I will have a small slice and feel grateful for the generosity of people. But because my general diet is devoid of hydrogenated fat the occasional instance of shortening will have no impact. The same is true for high fructose corn syrup. See Chapters 8-10 for help determining which foods to use as daily fuel and which foods are to be enjoyed only occasionally. The recipes at the end of this book bear an icon indicating whether I recommend them as daily fuel ✑ or as an occasional treat ♣.

Grace Period

In general, it takes about three days for exercise and diet to show up on your body. If you are leaner today, you can trace the effect to your activity and diet three days ago. So, you have a grace period. Don't ever derail your pursuit of good health by beating yourself up over the cookies, tacos, and ice cream you ate yesterday. You have at least two days to counter those food choices. In fact, the hallmark of a healthy metabolism is to enjoy Thanksgiving dinner (and the after-dinner turkey sandwiches) by getting up the next day in a healthy frame of mind ready to exercise and fulfill your body's requests for fuel. Simply return to your healthy habits and Thanksgiving dinner will make very little impact. I know I have said it before, but I will share it once again: It is what we do most regularly that determines how we look and feel.

The goal is to speed up your metabolism. The key is balance. The formula: moderate and consistent exercise blended with a diet of balanced foods. Voila!

By now you've probably noticed *Miracle Pill* is anathema to all diet programs because it changes thought paradigms from "immediate results" to "permanent behavior changes." The pursuit of health encourages long-range thinking and lifestyle adjustment. Whereas, diets are inherently short-term.

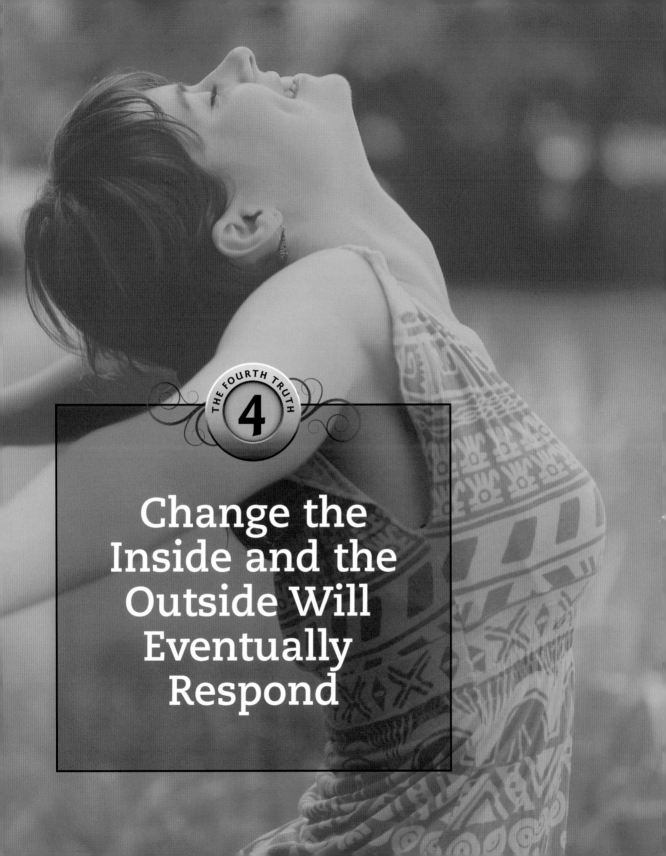

Change the Inside and the Outside Will Eventually Respond

Please take a moment to list up to 10 of your *best* physical features.

Top 10 Features

1 _____

2 _____

3 _____

4 _____

5 _____

6 _____

7 _____

8 _____

9 _____

10 _____

Now list up to 10 of your *worst* features (or body flaws).

10 Worst Features

1 _____

2 _____

3 _____

4 _____

5 _____

6 _____

7 _____

8 _____

9 _____

10 _____

First, decide which items on your "worst" list you have control over. Put a star by those items. For instance, you might put a star by hair color, stomach paunch, chewed fingernails, etc. Do not put a star by items out of your control such as ugly feet, skin blemishes, spider veins, cellulite, wrinkles, narrow shoulders, baldness, or big nose. Be realistic. Features that could be improved with surgical "freshening up" do not count as items "within your control"; they should *not* have a star by them. The following section deals with making peace with those parts that are outside of our control.

Second, compare lists. Which is longer? If your "worst" list is longer than your "best" list, you are pretty normal. Most of us self-critique our bodies pretty harshly. It is easier to acknowledge our flaws than our finer attributes. However, when we focus on our faults, we cannot feel gratitude for great features that came with our awesome machines. Take a moment to appreciate your stuff. Look at that "best features" list. What else belongs on that list? Keep going until you fill all 10 spots and then, if you wish, keep going.

Third, give yourself permission to make peace with those attributes on the second list that do not have a star by them (those features outside of your control). Don't hate those parts or wish them away. It is a giant waste of energy to obsess about wide hips and narrow lips. These are the body parts God intended for you to have. Do not feel intolerant of something you cannot do anything about. Your body is a Ferrari™. Please remember His design of your equipment included those features. It is the asymmetry of Mona Lisa's face that makes her so captivating.

> Courage, faith, and compassion are not only to be exercised on other people. Practice those qualities on yourself.

As you review your lists, be aware your features with a star by them will improve as you become a healthier manager of your body. That stomach paunch will certainly flatten out. Even hair, although not likely to change color without the help of hair dye, will, with increased health, become shinier and fuller. Be tolerant of yourself. Stay the course and changes will come. Courage, faith, and compassion are not only to be exercised on other people. Practice those qualities on yourself. When you have extended more grace to yourself, take the next step toward owning your situation, whether good or bad. This next section deals with taking responsibility for your choices. As you read, please maintain a spirit of compassion for all your qualities—self-acceptance empowers like nothing else.

Own Your Life

People do what they really want (in their hearts) to do. They go where they really want to go.

They choose people they really want to be around, etc. This is because we exist where we are most comfortable. In other words, responsibility for the quality of our lives is squarely on our own shoulders because we choose it.

People complain that they don't have the spouse they want, they are addicted to something and cannot quit, their job is too stressful, they don't make enough money, or they don't live where they want. But, in fact, with certain exceptions (like children born into war-ravaged countries) we are all exactly where we have chosen to be—although it may not be where we imagine we would be happiest. The good news: just as we have the power to create the life we are now living, we also have the power to create a different life—a fulfilled, happy, meaningful, abundant life. This is an empowering concept. As you own the life you live today, you become poised to move in a new direction, one that leads to the life that makes you happy.

Direction

I believe happiness is based more on the direction of the journey than the final destination. Choose your direction and live your life headed toward it. If you want to end up at point A, you cannot continue behaviors that head toward point B. For instance, if you want to be an energetic Grandfather for your grandchildren, you cannot spend most of your time sitting on the couch ignoring the grandkids.

I know a man who desperately wants a wife and family. He is successful, good-looking, intelligent, educated, and excellent with children. Yet he continues to live the life of a bachelor. He gravitates toward women who have not prepared themselves for the commitment of marriage. He spends a lot of time partying instead of positioning himself to meet the love of his life. He remains in relationships that are inconsistent with his goal. He is directionally challenged.

Set a course of action for where you want to be. If you want greater health, use the exercises and ideas in this book to improve your health. If you want to be happily married, figure out how to get there. If you want more money, make a plan. There will be bumps along the way and things might not go as predicted, but to end up at a certain point, we must travel in the direction leading to that point—and as a bonus, merely traveling in our desired direction makes us happy. Making excuses will not position you closer to your goal. Do not be directionally challenged.

The beauty of this life is we only need to live today. We don't need to worry about running out of motivation for tomorrow. Let tomorrow take care of itself. Live today a life that brings you closer to your goals. Tomorrow, wake up and do it again.

Not all goals are achievable nor should they be. Some pursuits are discovered to be undesirable only when we start working toward them; stay flexible with your goals. As a chef, I know a number of professionals who stepped into a culinary career quite late in life after they had built stellar careers in other industries. They were good at the other jobs, but cooking made them happy. These discoveries are gifts. Make a course correction when life teaches you to go in that new direction. If you have always thought you would be good at scrap-booking, but found it actually makes you anxious, change your plan. Discover something else that brings you peace. Even if you come from a long line of venerable scrap-bookers and "scrapping" is part of the local culture, shake off obligatory expectations and find the activities that match the gifts God sent you. Set your goals, whether they be career, hobby, health, or anything else, based on the direction you want to go and move forward. As long as your thoughts and behaviors are aligned with your goals, you will be fulfilled and true to yourself. The next section shatters the paradigm of thinking you are trapped in your situation and opens possible routes to your goals.

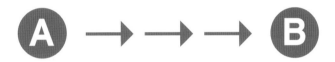

You Are Not Stuck

When you say, "I can't change, this is who I am," you are ignoring the gift of choice you have been given. You are who you decide to be. You are not stuck. Whether the issue is the condition of your body, marriage, job, family, or anything else, the principle remains true. Even a single mother raising children by herself is not stuck in her challenging situation. She is choosing to stick around for her kids. Taking the moral high ground and doing the right thing is absolutely a choice, even when it is exhausting and difficult. Think about it: if we were com-

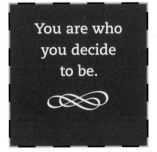

pelled by some unseen external force to always make the right choice, it would deny us the satisfaction, personal growth, and happiness that comes from *choosing* to do the right thing. Embracing our power of agency to make choices, even hard ones, develops our souls and helps us progress. Don't spend one minute floundering in the gray area of doing something because you are "supposed to" or "have to." Take ownership of your choices, identify those you want to change, and move forward.

Map Your Life

What direction do you want to go? Use the following pages to log in your desired destinations. There are four main areas for you to map:

1 Physical Mapping

2 Spiritual Mapping

3 Emotional Mapping

4 Intellectual Mapping

In each section describe in detail the destinations you want. Identify all the specifics you can. How does it feel? What does it look like? Why do you want it? How are you different with this change in your life? Use present-tense language when thinking this over. For instance, instead of thinking, "How *would I* be different?" contemplate, "How *am I* different?" Present tense imagery predicts truer results and prevents us from over or under inflating the value of a goal. Finally, list the steps you need to take to get to your desired destinations. This is more than a goal-setting activity—it can help you flesh out a complete picture of your ideal self and the changes needed to accomplish it. If you find you need more space continue on a separate paper or in a journal.

Physical Mapping

Decide how you want to feel and look. Be specific. Decide what abilities you want to possess. Do you want to walk up the stairs without your heart pounding? Make it a destination. Do you want to dance without your feet hurting? Make it a destination. Do you want to carry your child or grandchild without your back aching? I know it is tempting to start mapping the physical by scripting how you want to look, but resist making appearance the first thing on you map. How we look is important, but good looks start with health and health is akin to how you feel. Be reasonable. Don't waste time charting a goal of having long legs if you are five feet tall. However, you can choose to have strong sleek legs at any height. Some of the most gorgeous dancers in the world are short and they have legs to die for.

After deciding how you want to feel, and you get to the part where you decide how you want to look, please do it with self-love, not self-loathing. God did not make a mistake with you. Be filled with gratitude. There is nothing so sexy as a man or woman who feels confident in their own skin. I will never look like a super model and that is just fine. Super models will never look like me. Also fine. My nose looks like my father's. I have my mother's smile. Our physical features connect us to the people we came from. I will not insult my ancestors by degrading my forehead, thighs, chin, etc. Their lives were not dismissed because they fell short of some cultural notion of ideal beauty; neither will my life be meaningless if I don't look like a magazine cover. Within my control, I have a healthy strong body and a spirit filled with love. Can I manage my body so I fulfill my potential? Absolutely!

Use these pages to begin mapping your ideal physical self.

- ✖ How do you want to feel? List them all.
- ✖ Why do you want it?
- ✖ How are you different with this change in your life?
- ✖ How do you want to look?

_____

_____

_____

_____

_____

_____

_____

_____

Spiritual Mapping

This important category is often overlooked. Give yourself permission to enjoy the quiet peace resulting from a fulfilling spiritual life. Even if you have never given much veracity to spiritual concepts, indulge in the possibility of transcendent love and eternal purpose. The world does not trumpet the joys of faith and morality, but many happy people do. Map your pathway to a closer connection with God. List the behaviors and attitudes that bring you closer to Him. Perhaps prayer is a good way to feel a connection with Him. Because He created you and loves you, it makes sense that He might want to hear from you now and then. What other ways of growing spiritually interest you? Map them all.

Use these pages to map your ideal spiritual destination.

_____

_____

_____

_____

_____

_____

_____

_____

Emotional Mapping

How does one map an emotional destination? Consider first if you really take responsibility for your life. Many mistakes come from not developing emotional maturity. Whether emotional immaturity is the result of a bad childhood or bad character, you have the freedom to grow into an emotionally healthy person—if you map that course. For instance, if you are proud, list specific ways to be humble. If you are in denial, make honesty a practice. If you are selfish, chart a course towards caring for others, including unselfish service in your regular activities. Nothing generates gratitude and perspective like volunteering in the cancer wing of a children's hospital. Are you weak, angry, bitter, jealous, or petty? Many attitudes and habits that make us unhealthy stem from allowing our emotional growth to remain stunted. Do you tend to allow fear to disable you? Do you play the victim to avoid culpability? Are you a martyr—which is selfishness at its core? Here is a big one: do you occupy time with busyness as an excuse to avoid important things?

Take an honest inventory of how _you_ contribute to your relationships. Why have you made them what they are? Think about how you see food. Why have you decided to think about food and exercise the way you have? How do the roles you play in your family contribute to your healthy and unhealthy habits? These are deep questions and should not be glossed over. Take some time to complete your inventory and then make an action list of how you will proceed to align your emotions with your goals.

- Record an inventory of your emotional maturity and those things that need work.

- Consider your contribution to your relationships—what can you change?

- Own up to your attitudes about food and exercise.

List them all with new destinations and courses of action.

_____

_____

_____

_____

_____

_____

_____

_____

_____

_____

Intellectual Mapping

Decide which aspects of your intellect need improvement. Even super smart people get complacent now and then and need to be challenged. List the specific actions necessary to propel you in that direction. Improving your intellect is about progress, not winning or failing. Consider goals both large and small. Even small changes can be catalysts for great things. One day my sweet husband picked up _The Hobbit_, by J.R.R. Tolkein, and started to read. He was in his 30's and had not read a book since high school. Now in his mid-forties, he still reads every day. As a result of his reading habit, he finished his degree, started several new businesses, and increased his ability to learn. Einstein reportedly said the fastest way to become intelligent is to read. Whatever your intellectual destination, describe it in detail and figure out how to get there.

To help you get started, here are some possible destinations: Do you want to finish that degree? Have you always wanted to be fluent in Spanish? Have your kids surpassed you in math because you forgot algebra? Do you need to learn certain computer skills to make more money at work? Is there a career you want but have avoided because it required certification and knowledge you just don't have? Have you read a book in the last 30 days (other than this one)? Can you articulate your point in a two-sided debate? Can you problem solve in a rational, unemotional manner (this means getting out of the airport parking lot without a flare, compass, and a GPS)?

Use these pages to map your intellectual destination.

_____

_____

_____

_____

_____

_____

_____

Payoff

While we are taking responsibility for our situations, let's talk about payoff. Although our choices may not make us happy, there is some kind of payoff in every choice. To be clear, payoff is different from consequence. For instance, the *consequence* of driving too fast may be a speeding ticket. The *payoff* for driving too fast is the exhilaration of speed and the thrill of risky behavior. We don't always get to choose consequences. But payoff is the real motivation behind the action and we definitely choose our payoffs. Consequences can be pleasant or unpleasant, whereas payoffs, or the true objects of our pursuit, are desirable.

If we struggle with consistent exercise and healthy food, it may be that those behaviors don't present an enticing enough payoff for us. One could argue, *"I don't like feeling fat and unhealthy. I hate the feeling I get from bingeing on cold cereal late at night. There's no payoff in that!"*

Well, actually, we do like it on some level. When we pursue a behavior not in line with our goals, we do so because it promises a tastier payoff. Only when we accept this fact can we make a change. We might not be at our high school weight, but the payoff for staying fat is, in some ways, more comfortable. What possible payoffs could there be for staying fat? Keep reading to discover your personal answer.

Payoffs for NOT Exercising

There are all kinds of payoffs for not exercising. Perhaps we feel rebellious. Like a three-year old, we brace ourselves, squint our eyes, and say, "No, I won't!" Or, we feel ambivalence or contempt. We might even define "taking care of ourselves" as pampering in the form of sitting around, which makes getting up and going for a run feels like a chore. No one wants another chore, so a preference for sedentary self-care results in a life without regular exercise.

If the following examples do not include your payoffs, truthfully figure out what yours are in the payoff exercise that follows.

Other Payoff Examples:

1 What are the payoffs for an alcoholic? They might include escape from reality and responsibility (through a form of self-medication), the general numbing of emotions, narcissism, withdrawal from other people, hedonistic pleasure, etc.

2 What is the payoff for serving our families (bandaging scrapes, bringing home a paycheck, helping with homework, cooking, cleaning, mowing the lawn, carpooling the soccer

team, driving to and from clarinet lessons, etc.)? Payoffs could include satisfaction, martyrdom, fulfillment, building bonds of love, or even possibly avoiding taking care of ourselves.

3   What is the payoff for eating a double serving of dinner? Perhaps extended time at the table, a desire to prevent wasted food, an attempt to make the work of preparing the meal more meaningful—you liked it enough to have seconds, or maybe we keep on eating to escape from emotions.

4   What is the payoff for joining a co-ed volleyball league? It might include the thrill of competition, a desire to feel young and vital, the hope of a love connection, added exercise in your week, the healthy catharsis of hitting a volleyball instead of your boss, the satisfaction of improving athletic skills, or an escape from the thoughts normally occupying your mind.

Bulimia and My Crazy Payoffs

As evidence that even the most painful conditions can be perpetuated due to payoffs, I want to share my struggle and eventual triumph over bulimia. From the time I was thirteen years old until my early twenties, I experienced bulimic compulsions. Here is how it would present: After a stressful day, I would find a quiet place to zone-out in front of the television and binge on a whole pint of ice cream. Then the ice cream would be followed by a purge of the contents of my swollen belly into the toilet. The turning point came one night when I dreaded, more than usual, the drained, nauseated feeling I would inevitably experience after the purge. Although I had just consumed massive quantities of food, I knew the relief and euphoria that always accompanied the purge would be dwarfed by the disgust, shame, and fear that came with it. I found myself examining the payoffs of this dangerous habit.

I made the decision to resist the urge to purge. I cried myself to sleep that night convinced I would be fat and unlovable forever. The next day I forced myself to exercise moderately and eat sensibly. I felt a little better. When the temptation to binge came again the next day, I thought about the unappealing payoffs of the purge—and I resisted. I kept resisting. After a few months, the urge to binge tempted me only occasionally. After a few years, it went away almost entirely.

Looking back, I see why I stopped my bulimic binges: I wanted health more than I wanted the relief,

*Many eating disorders require the professional help of a physician or psychiatrist. If you struggle with these issues, please immediately seek help from a doctor or an experienced specialist in eating disorders.

the false sense of control, and the escape of binge and purge. The payoff for quitting this habit was a sense of accomplishment and a foundation for moderate eating. Self-mastery was possible. I still wasn't healthy, but at least I was not a slave to bulimic cravings. I no longer kept a dark secret. The vomit-induced sore throat and acid reflux went away. My complexion cleared up. I no longer had to be embarrassed about spending so much time in the bathroom after a big meal. The payoffs were simply better. It was an empowering lesson to learn, the benefits of which have generalized to all aspects of my life.

Your Payoffs

This next section requires brutally honest introspection regarding your payoffs. While doing this exercise, decide what you get from *not* taking care of yourself inside and out.

It might be painful, but we certainly don't fool anyone by cheating. We only stunt our own progress by evading the truth. Besides, the world sees our struggle with weight because we wear it on the outside. Be honest to move forward.

List 10 behaviors that you want to change or eliminate, identifying their corresponding payoffs.

Your Payoffs – List 1

OLD BEHAVIORS & ATTITUDES   PAYOFFS

1 _____   _____

_____   _____

2 _____   _____

_____   _____

3 _____   _____

_____   _____

4 _____   _____

_____   _____

5 _____   _____
   _____   _____

6 _____   _____
   _____   _____

7 _____   _____
   _____   _____

8 _____   _____
   _____   _____

9 _____   _____
   _____   _____

10 _____   _____
   _____   _____

List 10 new behaviors (or attitudes), and list their corresponding payoffs.

Your Payoffs – List 2

NEW BEHAVIORS & ATTITUDES   PAYOFFS

1 _____   _____
   _____   _____

2 _____   _____
   _____   _____

3 _____   _____
   _____   _____

4 _____   _____
   _____   _____

5 _____   _____
   _____   _____

6 _____   _____
   _____   _____

7 _____   _____
   _____   _____

8 _____   _____
   _____   _____

9 _____   _____
   _____   _____

10 _____   _____
   _____   _____

Now examine your lists. Do you want the new payoffs more than the old payoffs? How badly?

TIP 5

"Do I want this handful of chips more than I want to reach my goal?" Compulsive eating, or rather, nervous and distracted eating, can be squelched by repeatedly asking yourself the direct question: "Do I want this (fill in the blank) more than I want to be at a healthy weight?" Be honest and give yourself an answer. Sometimes, the answer is yes. Chocolate can be medicinal. But when extra slices of buttered bread start shouting at you to eat them, and you do not need them at that moment, fall back on this private conversation with yourself. With every declination, you empower yourself and further alter your habits.

Change the Inside

To change the outside forever, begin to change the inside. Just like the case of teenage acne that requires more than a dab of over-the-counter acne lotion, the major healing comes from fixing the problem from the inside. It is only when we change who we are on the inside—change how we think, what we want, and how we live—that we see permanent results.

But, When Will I See Change?

Three months into my process, I hit a low point. The thrill of newly purchased stretchy pants and sexy work out videos was gone. I had diligently logged in 45-minute workouts six times per week, and I should have been losing weight. But, I could see no visible change and my clothes fit the same. And then to make matters worse, the scale informed me I had not lost even one single pound of fat. In a state of dejection, I considered giving up and resigning myself to being fat. I cried for a day.

It was during this despondent crisis that I had another self-actualization moment. I realized I could either stop my exercise program, which was justified considering the time and effort involved, or continue exercising. I begrudgingly decided to keep sweating, even if it never shaved off the weight, because I knew exercise was good for me and I felt a responsibility to model a healthy lifestyle for my daughter.

I kept at it, and three months later, I noticed an interesting thing. My pants fit looser. My thighs looked less wobbly. My back ached less. By golly, I was losing weight! It took SIX MONTHS for my body to begin using fat for fuel, but eventually, my metabolism ramped up and I enjoyed steady weight loss for the next three years. By steady, I mean about 2-3 pounds a month.

If 2-3 pounds a month seems slow, remember, the slower it comes off, the easier it stays off. I was not interested in buying a "quick" diet program only to find myself dieting again six months later. I wanted to get to a healthy weight and stay there indefinitely. Intuitively, I knew this slow, healthy change in my body would help me achieve permanent health and beauty. You know it, too.

So, when will you see change? It depends on many factors, but certainly it will take time for your metabolism to change. It took about six months for my fat cells to release fat for fuel while I was exercising. It could take much less for you. But, once my body learned to use up excess fat stores, it continued to burn fat—because I continued to exercise daily and place a demand on my body.

Male bodies typically respond to exercise faster, sometimes in only a in a matter of days. Some women over forty will need to be consistent for months before their metabolisms respond. Ladies, don't whine about the injustice, just focus on your goal. Regardless of how long it takes for you, stick with it. I find it encouraging that I have within my control the ability to make my body perform in my favor. Remember, you become healthier when you exercise (even if you never lose a pound), than if you were inactive. So really, by exercising, you have nothing to lose—but fat.

The Inside Had Changed

It took me almost four years to lose over 100 pounds—which was exactly the amount of time my body needed. I maintained this healthy weight for two years and then I was blessed with another pregnancy. Although I was thrilled to be pregnant, I was also scared of becoming fat.

I had a few surprises in store for me. During the pregnancy, I continued to want exercise and healthy food just as I had before. Despite nausea and weight gain, my lifestyle choices remained pretty much what they were before. Because the baby was in the captain's chair, accommodations were made—a second breakfast and third dinner were required for my body to build a new little person. Still, I did my best. I gained a total of 55-pounds (quite reasonable for me) and delivered a healthy baby boy. The birth was accomplished in about 20 minutes without the use of drugs. Furthermore, after the birth, I resumed the same healthy habits as before the pregnancy. I did not revert back to the mind-set of the fat person I had been before. I was changed on the inside.

After childbirth without dieting or restricting myself, I quickly lost the baby weight and went on to have a third child with the same healthy result. Now, over 15-years later, I have maintained a healthy body. I will never go back to being the person I was before because I am changed on the inside. I now think like a healthy, fit person and I act like a healthy, fit person. I shop and eat and play like a...you know the rest. It would be impossible for me to go back to being the unbalanced fat girl I was before due to the fact that the payoff is simply better with health. I have new habits. My pants fit, and I have the energy to teach my kids to do flips on the trampoline—*that* is my payoff.

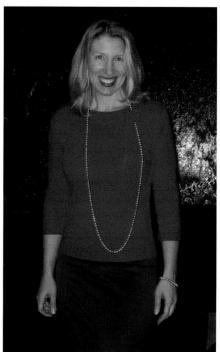

PHOTO: JON HATCH

Here I am at age 39, after 13-years, 3 babies, and, ultimately, 110-pounds of weight loss.

Commitment

It is impossible to become committed wholly to something unless we are actively doing it. "Theoretical" exercise does not burn "actual" fat. The mental shift from wishing to doing only happens after we "do" long enough for a new habit to form.

> The mental shift
> from wishing to
> doing only happens
> after we "do" long
> enough for a new
> habit to form.

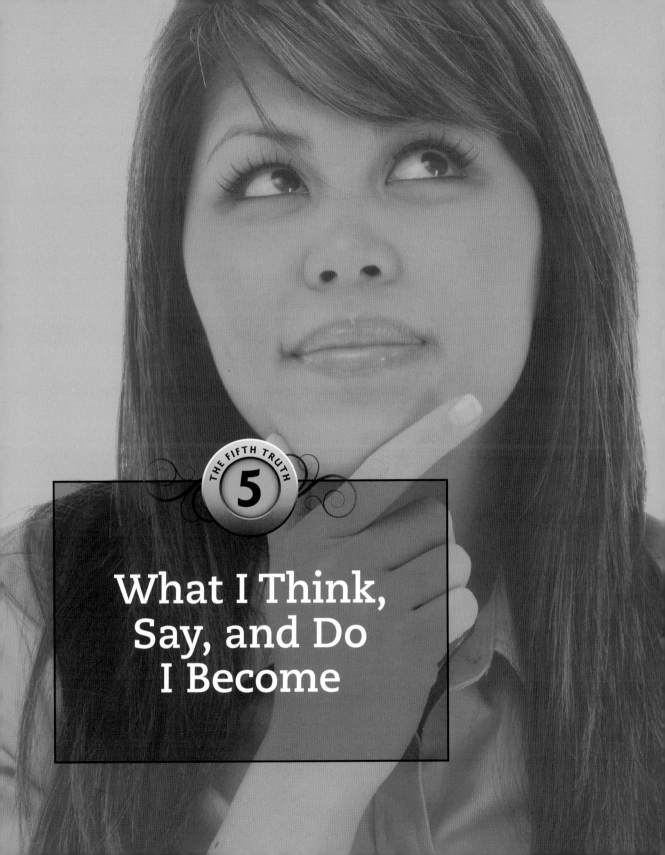

What I Think, Say, and Do I Become

This chapter is all about self-actualization and to that end—change. Why is it so hard to change our thinking and how do we make it permanent? The answers to these questions are discussed below. This first section helps us see ourselves in a different light. The second section reveals scientific evidence of the truth: "What I Think, Say, and Do, I Become." The rest of the chapter deals with habits we presently have, how habits can become permanently changed, and techniques for making these changes.

Your mapping work in the previous chapter should have clarified your vision of who you want to be. Your efforts to realize the new "you" may have already begun. Use the ideas in this chapter to springboard into new habits.

Mortal Bodies

I love my body. I believe it is a gift from God. In the Apostle Paul's ancient epistle to the Corinthians, he defined our bodies as sacred temples because they contain holy spirits—namely ours. (*1 Corinthians 3:16*) Our spirits are holy because we are the literal spirit sons and daughters of The Father, who is holy. A temple can be any place where a holy spirit dwells. Therefore, our bodies are holy temples.

I believe we show respect for our Heavenly Father by managing our bodies well. If you were the sole caretaker of a sacred building, would you allow it to fall into a state of disrepair? Would you neglect the grounds until they were overrun with weeds? Would you allow anything within its holy walls that was not clean and pure? You are the steward of your mortal temple. The way you manage this *house* reflects the respect you have for your spirit.

From this perspective, I will never hate my body again. I will only treat it with the utmost care. I wake up each morning and say a silent "thank you" and list all the things for which I am grateful, including my body. As age changes my body, I trust the aging process is part of the design of mortality. No botox or freshening up is required. I have earned every wrinkle and varicose vein by living the life I chose. My Heavenly Father gave me the gifts of my life and body. I trust Him enough to believe the challenges of age are necessary requirements for my ultimate progress and learning.

Thought Power

Thoughts carry energy. New technologies now enable scientists to see and measure the shift in energy when we focus our thoughts from one thing to the next. High tech equipment reveals this energy is not just contained within the sphere of our heads, it projects beyond our bodies—out into the universe. Our attitudes, feelings, and thoughts impact our lives and, as measurable energy, the lives of everyone around us.

On the subject of "thought-power," there is a great deal of medical knowledge the scientific community is only just beginning to grasp. For instance, traditional Asian medicine has five thousand years of wisdom treating energy imbalance (remember, thoughts have energy). This ancient art recognizes our thoughts and feelings have a direct impact on our health. More and more throughout the world, science is beginning to acknowledge the inseparable connection between mind and body. We know stress creates a negative impact on health. Inversely, we know positive thinking is a powerful tool for healing. The following section contains medical findings that prove it is possible to re-program our brains for a desired outcome.

Wiring Our Brains

We can change the wiring of our brains based on our thoughts and experiences. Doctors have long known our brains have the ability to re-wire and re-route around damaged or diseased areas. For example, in many cases stroke victims can learn to walk and talk again after experiencing brain damage. However, it was not until more advanced scanning equipment enabled us to "see" into the brain that we have begun to understand how this works. One exciting result of these findings is the degree to which our brains physically change when they are exposed to any input, whether compensating for damage or accommodating new information. We really do create ourselves by what we think, say, and do. The notion we come to this life with set talents, proclivities, and intelligence, without the real ability to change our thinking patterns, is dispelled as researches make advancements in the science of mapping the human brain. We can permanently change the way we think about food and exercise, based on healthy/positive input we give ourselves regarding food and exercise.

The following studies are evidence of our ability to change how we think on a profoundly biological level:

Rutgars University researcher and noted neuroscientist Paula Tallal found brain growth and greater synaptic activity by exposing dyslexic students to software designed to help them perceive sounds in a more "normal" way. As they received healthy stimulus, the size of the student's brains actually grew in response to learning! According to Tallal, "You create your brain from the input you get." (*Paula Tallal, 81-84*).

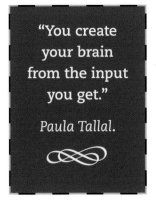

"You create your brain from the input you get."

Paula Tallal.

In another study, subjects were scanned after learning a simple piano exercise. Led by Dr. Alvaro Pascual-Leone at Harvard University, this study's results showed the brain motor cortex had changed as a direct result of their piano practice.

Interestingly, a separate group experienced an equally pronounced change despite the fact that they learned the piano exercise without actually moving their hands, but rather by only thinking about doing it (*A. Pascual-Leone, 315-329*).

The phenomenon of memory is also the result of measurable synaptic change caused by encoding our neurons with stimulation. Here's how memory works: after hearing the theme song to a new TV show, the connections in your brain display a teensy bit of growth. This growth represents a single exposure to the theme song or short-term memory. But short-term memory changes last only for a few minutes. Without repeated exposure, within 45 minutes the configuration of the brain returns to its previous state which is why you cannot remember the theme song a week later. However, after multiple stimulations over the course of an hour, such as hearing the theme song over and over, synapses take on a permanent change that will last a lifetime. This is long-term memory (*M.A. Colicos, 605-615*).

Clearly, a cheetah can change its spots. Science supports the fact that as new input, external or imagined, is repeatedly introduced, pathways in the brain become changed. Repeat a new action or thought enough times and these changes become permanent. To put this in context with weight loss, if I think I am a thin person, my brain will re-wire to process thoughts permanently like a thin person. Hence, I will behave like a thin person, and accordingly, take on the shape of a thin person.

Eliminate Evil Talking In My Head

The first implement of change is the elimination of negative speaking—to ourselves. If you have this habit, change it today by replacing thoughts of self-criticism, guilt, and self-hate, with gratitude and optimism. Things I formerly said to myself were loathsome and literally poisonous. As I derided myself with names like "fat pig," and "disgusting," I merely reinforced again and again that I would behave like a fat pig and be disgusting. My negative thoughts made it very difficult to see myself from a healthy perspective and, therefore, act like a healthy person.

How do we become a healthy person on the inside? Begin each day with thoughts of gratitude for your magnificent body. Nowhere is there a more resplendent manifestation of God's love for His children than the bodies he blessed us with. They cannot be duplicated. They are self-healing, opposable-thumb bearing, water-resistant, ambulatory wonders. Nothing can compare to the human form for beauty and function. Make these grateful thoughts innate by expressing them in a prayer of thanks or a meditation of gratitude.

Dissatisfaction with your body can hinder gratitude. Whether healthy or disabled, old or young, big or small, hairy or smooth, we can find endless points for which to be grateful. If your teeth have fallen out, be grateful for your elbows and their incredible hinges. If your toenails have fungus, be grateful for your ears that can hear someone say, "I love you." A stomach need not be flat and firm for us to be grateful for the healthy digestion which goes on inside. My Mom always said, *"If you can take food in one end and get rid of it out of the other, be grateful—you are healthy."* If confined to a chair, be grateful for a mind and soul that can soar with the joy of gratitude. *Happy* heals better than sad—and it sure is more fun!

It Takes Courage to Lose Weight

Following gastric bypass surgery, my dear college friend experienced fear after losing 30-pounds. She felt anxiety about further weight loss because the drastic changes in her body would undoubtedly facilitate the need for a new identity. Those who have never been fat do not understand the very real conundrum she faced as she anticipated becoming a thin person for the first time in her life. She feared she would not know the new woman in the mirror. She asked me, *"Who will I be when I am thin?"*

A lot is revealed about ourselves when we lose weight. Our personal power increases. The angles of our faces start to appear. The contours of our bodies are revealed. Our profile in its true form becomes apparent for the world, and ourselves, to see. Old aches and pains go away. Our energy patterns change, meaning our capabilities increase. We can do more and, therefore, we become more powerful in the world. This can cause anxiety for anyone who has hid behind fat for any amount of time.

It takes courage to brave uncharted waters and unfold day-by-day the new person you will become. Self-love should reflect the essence of who you are, not your dress size. It is the constant in your changeable world. Hold on to your positive, grateful outlook and you will emerge as a stronger, more empowered person. Do not let fear prevail. Ultimately, those who master themselves can master anything, meaning the pursuit of balance is worth feeling uncomfortable with the new you.

Installing New Habits

Installing new habits takes time for repetition and reinforcement. It is commonly said that it takes 21 days to make a new habit and 3 days to break it. These guidelines may or may not apply to you. Any smoker who quits will tell you it can take a lot longer than 21 days to become a non-smoker in their minds. I know people who still dream about cigarettes after ten years of abstinence. Don't despair; taking on a new healthy identity may require less time. There are people who make such a profound mental switch to non-smoking that cold turkey really means cold turkey. Your switch to health can be just as immediate.

You will discover how long it will take for you to wake up with a new desire to eat the right fuel and exercise moderately. Should you wake up and think, *(Groan!) When am I going to go for my run today?*—hurray! You now exercise consistently enough to plan it the moment you wake up. This is a good thing because it proves you established a new habit. The groan is ok. Reluctance is natural because exercise takes effort and maybe you don't love it yet—but you will. Reluctance does not need to keep you from becoming a consistently active person. Only when you push exercise out of your schedule until there is simply no time left in the day, will reluctance make you fail.

Installing new habits applies to food as well as exercise. The next time you pull through the fast food drive-thru and opt for the salad, congratulate yourself on reinforcing your new habit. It takes time and consistency to transition a diet from unbalanced to balanced because our menu choices are largely habit-driven. Fresh salads, whole grains, legumes, fruits, and lean meats taste better after a few weeks of choosing them. Drinking water instead of coffee or soda is a habit. Choosing a turkey sandwich on whole grain bread instead of a burger is as much a habit as is anything else we do.

Eating out at restaurants can derail even the most dedicated. Carefully own your menu choices. When I go to a steakhouse, I don't order a steak unless that is what my body really needs (which only happens during the coldest months of winter and after strenuous physical activity). Most of the time, I order salad, chicken, or fish. Whatever menu item suits my needs becomes my meal. Just as a cool glass of water tastes best when I am thirsty, the supercharged fuel of grilled Portobello mushrooms, zucchini, eggplant, and onions with barbecue sauce, when my body needs it, tastes better than a steak with fries.

I find it is easier to fuel my body correctly when I eat the majority of my meals at home. Eating from home gives me control over portion size and the amount of fat, sugar, and processing in my food. Despite my experience as a chef, at home I enjoy simply-prepared food based on the things my body needs. It is not unusual for me to serve roasted fish, steamed broccoli, and brown rice with a drizzle of soy sauce. Food doesn't need a fancy name or complicated composition to taste wonderful. Food in its purest form fulfills my nutritional needs and tastes good. Homemade granola with skim milk starts my day with serious high-protein fuel. I usually want a salad or sandwich with lean protein for lunch. Yes, I put mayonnaise on my sandwich and loads of creamy dressing on my salads. I enjoy a drizzle of olive oil on my pasta and a pat of butter on my fish. I am not on a diet. I do opt to live healthy, with a healthy

> **Reluctance does not need to keep you from becoming a consistently active person.**
>
>

> **It is not our occasional treats that define our bodies—it is our regular food choices that determine how we look and feel.**
>
>

> *Nay-Sayers. Be cautious of placing too much emphasis on negative influences. People often claim they can't lose weight because of negativity from family members or spouses. Occasionally loved ones will be resistant to our changes. They may be comfortable with the way things are. Change may shake them up a little bit.*
>
> *Regardless, don't pay heed to the critics in your life or put too much investment behind their opinions. They will adapt because you are going to change whether they like it or not. Think about it this way: you are inevitably going to change in a multitude of ways over the course of your life, (gray hair, mellower attitude, new music preferences, etc.), so a healthier lifestyle is just one new aspect to you. Don't put a lot of emphasis on the attitudes of those around you. In truth, their power is only what you give them.*

amount of fats. Sure there are the occasional treats and splurges. I enjoy a good onion ring or a brownie as much as the next person. However, it is not our occasional treats that define our bodies—it is our regular food choices that determine how we look and feel.

Hazards

During this process of creating new habits there are plenty of obstacles to derail us. Becoming aware of these hazards makes it easier to sidestep them. Here are a few you might have encountered—I know I did:

- Mapping a course in the wrong direction
- Pay offs reinforcing the unwanted habit instead of the desired goal
- A negative self-paradigm (low self-esteem)
- Negative self-talk
- Poorly managing my time to prevent exercise and healthy eating
- Impatience with my exercise program—not waiting for my body to learn to use fat for fuel
- Listening to nay-sayers
- Habitual Investment (page 59)

Have Faith in Success

Sometimes we don't believe an exercise program will truly work for us: *"Sure exercise makes my sister thin, but it doesn't work for me."* Either we suspect we will ultimately sabotage our weight loss with food or we claim to be unaffected by exercise.

When we don't believe exercise will be successful, working out feels like we are *impersonating* the habits of a fit person—instead of *incorporating* the habits of a fit person. *Trust* in exercise and believe it will eventually result in a trimmer body—*for you*.

What we think, say, and do, we become. Imagine you have been a fit person for 20 years and behave as if you believe exercise is the formula for wearing sexy jeans. Once you become healthy and trim, you no longer need to have faith because at that point you already fit in those jeans. However, until you gain personal experience as a healthy person, suspend disbelief and keep exercising.

We Probably Already Know the Answer

"I have battled my weight for so long. I just don't know what to do!" Yes, you do. Haven't you intuitively known healthy food and regular exercise is the formula for a trim body? Maybe in the past you became side-tracked by effective marketing that baited you with "fast" results, but haven't you have always known the simple truth on a practical level? Don't waffle around with the excuse that you don't know what to do. Trust your instincts.

When we truly want to do the right thing, our minds know right from wrong. The course you should take is that familiar nagging voice in your head. Recognize untruths and excuses, and push them aside. Pursue the right thing, even if it is hard, and you will realize success in areas that have value.

TIP
7

The Secret. Read or watch **The Secret**, *by Rhonda Byrne, available in book or DVD formats. Despite its material acquisition rhetoric, it is an interesting examination of the relationship between our thoughts and our realities.*

Habitual Investment

Years ago a friend confided in me how baffled she was that she never could keep a consistent exercise regimen going. She claimed to enjoy exercising, but she would inevitably drop out of her routine. She felt disgust for her lack of tenacity.

We often blame a failed diet or exercise program on a lack of self-control. Instead, we may be experiencing a human tendency I like to call: "habitual investment," meaning we tend to do what we have done before because we are more comfortable and familiar with whatever we do repeatedly. We sometimes defend our preference for the familiar even if it doesn't make us happy. We become "invested," not necessarily because it is the best choice, but merely because it is the course we are accustomed to. You probably know the cliché, *"The devil you know is better than the devil you don't."* Well, instead of flogging ourselves for lack of discipline, we might figure out how invested we are in behaviors we want to change.

My friend realized the "dropping out" part of her exercise pattern was all too familiar. She was emotionally invested in *discontinuing* her exercise program. She started and stopped so many times she created a habit of stopping after a week or two. What she needed was to become invested in *consistent* exercise 5-6 times per week.

TIP 8

The key to a new habit is consistency, not intensity of desire.

The Default Setting

Except for those enlightened moments when we flip mental switches and install new actions in our life, such as those from the *Life Mapping* section of Chapter 4, we tend to make decisions on auto pilot mode. It can be helpful to recognize most of us have a default automatic setting for our daily routine. Surprisingly, in the average day we do not make many new choices. A large percentage of our day-to-day actions are the result of habit. We choose to live like this because it is easier and takes less energy to repeat a previous thought or action than to do things a new way every time. Think about your routine. Do you brush your teeth the same way every day? Do you answer the telephone the same way? Do you put your socks on the same way? Do you drive the same road to work every day?

There is no moral judgment (good or bad) attached to acting primarily out of habit.

We are creatures of habit. But, these same patterns apply to food choices. If you tend to grab a handful of cookies for a snack, even when you may really only want one (hey, it could happen), you will probably still eat a handful of cookies out of habit. You don't have to blame yourself as a gluttonous, non-disciplined cookie-monster. You are quite normal. If you always eat at bedtime, recognize that behavior as part of your default setting—a setting that can be changed with repetition of the new behavior. Because knowledge is power, become aware when your routine does not move you closer to your goals.

While changing the default setting, only create new behaviors that can be maintained for the rest of your life. If you don't like running, perhaps try yoga. If you don't like swimming, try dancing. Whatever you begin, make sure it is of moderate intensity so you can get up and do it again tomorrow. It does you no good to kill yourself in a marathon-training program for a few days only to quit because you are too sore and tired to continue. Aim for new activities

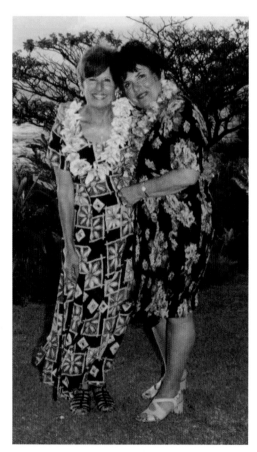

Irene (on right) "before," age 55

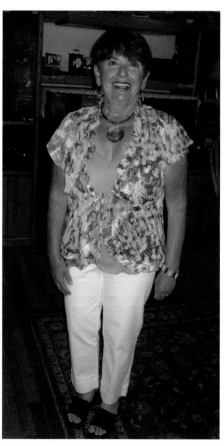

After 26-pounds of weight loss, age 65

you can carry into your 70's and 80's. See Chapters 6 and 7 for an in-depth examination of consistency.

My mother-in-law grew up in an era when women simply did not put on exercise clothes and work out. She started walking in her 50's. Daily exercise was new to her. Despite this, she persevered. After ten years of walking her dog every day, she added 5 minutes of running, at a very slow pace. She expanded that run to 20 minutes total—in the middle of her walk. She also started resistance training with weights to improve muscle tone and bone density. She is now 26 pounds lighter and has maintained her youthful figure for years. Even the dog is healthier. She credits Miracle Pill concepts, including consistent walking with a little running and resistance training for her transformation.

"Slow-and-steady wins-the-race" may not be a sexy marketing hook, but it is successful for weight management. Start activities that are comfortable, affordable, and can be continued for the rest of your life. Begin at a pace and level of intensity that challenges you, but does not leave you sore. Slowly increase duration and intensity, taking years to increase if necessary. Remember, if you become sore, you won't want to do it again tomorrow. Consistency will get you to your goal; too much intensity will make you ache. Resist the tendency to compete in some imaginary contest. I don't care how bouncy the other women in my aerobic class are. If I feel shoulder pain, it is not in my best interest to wave my arms about over my head. I modify the movement to receive the aerobic benefits and return tomorrow for another class.

Visualization

Pioneered decades ago as a way to improve athletic performance at a high level, visualization techniques are an effective way to produce results. Boiled down to the bare bones, visualization means you picture yourself experiencing whatever you want to accomplish, complete with the emotions you would have if experiencing it for real. For instance, a high jumper would visualize a successful jump from beginning to end. This exercise improves performance and helps create the desired outcome.

You can implement this practice in the pursuit of any goal—including body transformation. Start while in a focused, relaxed state. Fix a clear intention in your mind of what you want to happen and how you want to feel. For example, during the last ten minutes of a run, see a clear picture of your body in its ideal state: flat belly, trim hips, strong arms, straight spine. Picture your stride, lean muscles powering each step—no jiggle in your backyard, no thighs rubbing together. Infuse your mind with a grateful loving feeling toward your body, regardless whether this visualization matches reality or not. Visualization will help you realize the image in your head, but only if accompanied with positive enthusiasm for the process. You cannot bear resentment for your body and create a positive outcome (*A.R. Isaac, 192-198*).

Return to this visualization on a regular basis to speed your body to your desired state. Visualization is particularly effective when applied to physical endeavors, such as improving your golf swing, toning your body, and building endurance. It also produces psychological benefits (*K.A. Martin and C.R. Hall, 54-69*).

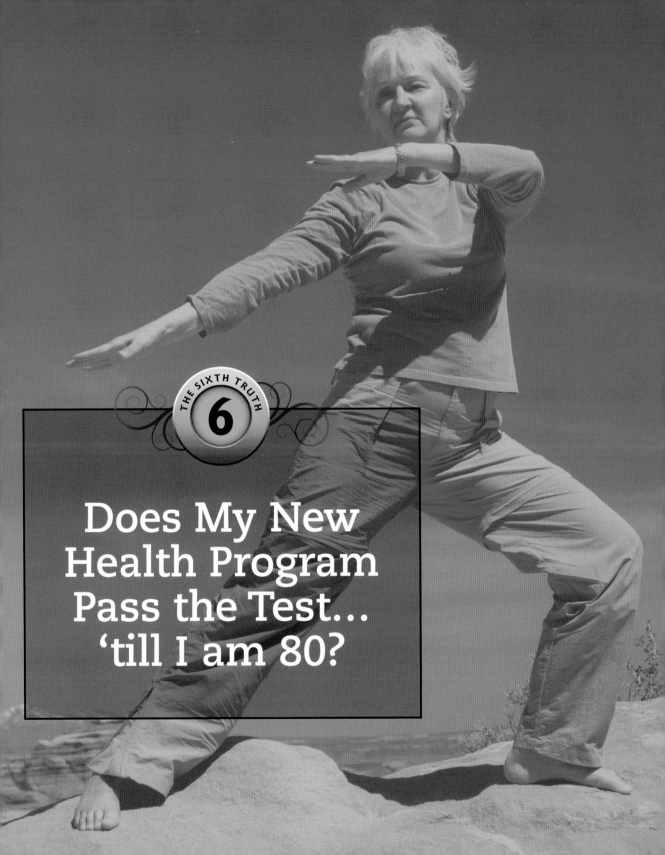

THE SIXTH TRUTH

6

Does My New
Health Program
Pass the Test...
'till I am 80?

Don't Buy Into the Wrong Ideal

Are you a "chronic" dieter? If not, you probably know someone who is. Chronic dieters are always trying one weight-loss program after another, but they never seem to keep weight off. For many it is an obsession. If you answered "yes," you are certainly not alone. On a grand societal scale, weight loss has become germane to the collective mentality of most developed countries. Here in the West losing weight appears to have become our national pastime. Even China, formerly comprised of entirely thin people, is experiencing an economic boost from the explosion of weight loss products and marketing. Yes, Chinese people are getting fat from the relatively new inclusion of sugar, greater quantities of meat (and food in general), and processed foods into their diets. These factors combined with the industrialization of jobs has begun to create more sedentary existences similar to those of other developed countries. Ironically, just 200 years ago, a little extra fat was a symbol of success. Throughout history, man's prosperity was recognized by extra girth around his or her middle. Now, with fairly inexpensive food available across all socio-economic lines, the poor have become fat and members of our well-heeled set claim status by becoming dangerously thin. One glance at magazine racks will tell you today's declaration of beauty is a minimal-sized body wearing minimal clothing.

I don't buy into the saying: "You can never be too thin." Nope. People really do come in all shapes and sizes and, with health, variations on "ideal" are all beautiful. Don't buy into a false premise. Your best self is the healthiest version of you. Period.

My body is a gift to me. If my higher power sees fit to bless me with the gift of mortality, I have a responsibility to appreciate it—warts and all, whether or not I am 5-foot-10-inches tall and wear a size 0. Change your ideal from looking like someone else to looking like a healthier version of you, without dieting. At the core of this chapter is the value of permanence.

Litmus Test

"Can I consistently maintain any new diet or exercise program until I am 80-years old, or older?"

According to the Merriam-Webster dictionary, litmus is a coloring agent derived from lichens that turns red in acid solutions and blue in alkaline—terribly useful in science. Like that unfailing color test, you can hold up any and all diet and exercise programs to the following question: "Can I consistently maintain it until I am 80-years old, or older?" If the answer is yes, it is a lifestyle change. If not, it is a quick fix and should be abandoned (unless you enjoy losing and re-losing the same fat over and over). I use the arbitrary age of eighty to illustrate the value of long-term behavioral adjustments—you could insert 108-years old if you wish.

As a result of this test, I refuse to begin a low carbohydrate diet because I cannot give up bread until I am eighty. A crusty slice of warm sourdough bread with a generous slather of butter is not something I will live without. Therefore, a bread-free diet is not a permanent lifestyle change and will only result in my feeling deprived and, quite frankly, grumpy.

I can, however, choose primarily whole-grain bread instead of white bread. I can also include one raw vegetable or fruit in each meal. I can replace processed meat like sausage and ham, or fatty meat like hamburger, with lean chicken, turkey, or fish. I can expand my grain intake to include brown rice, oatmeal, and alternative grains like quinoa, barley, and spelt. A smidge of butter or drizzle of good olive oil on top of those grains doesn't hurt my feelings either. Can I enjoy all these foods for the rest of my life? Absolutely! Will these adjustments make me feel deprived of tasty food? Never.

In terms of exercise, boot-camp style workouts lasting hours on-end are not sustainable and, for most people, neither are expensive health club memberships or personal trainers. On the other hand, a good pair of exercise shoes won't set you back too much and using them is free. Choose activities you can maintain for years to come. Cross training with a variety of activities helps work all your muscle groups. Try dancing, swimming, weight training, recreational sports like volleyball and softball, tennis, yoga, hiking, biking, etc.—all of which can be part of an active lifestyle for the rest of your life. Personally, I like to walk four times a week with about 20 minutes of slow running in the middle of the walk. I stretch after my run/walk using yoga breathing techniques. I also enjoy recreational volleyball twice a week along with a Latin-rhythm cardio class once a week. I love hiking, water sports, yoga, and any activity in general. It is not uncommon for me to round up the kids and take the family on a stroll. Sometimes my husband and I will go dancing for a date. I have found I feel better when I am in motion. Some people want to lie by a pool for vacation. My idea of relaxation is to move my body.

Several years ago, a friend invited me to train with her for a big national marathon. I asked her about the training requirements. As I listened to her describe the initial daily mileage of 6-8 miles I thought, "*Although that is double what I normally run, I could possibly do it for a month.*" Then she told me the mileage would need to increase to 10-12 miles a day, followed by three weeks of 16 mile runs. My eyes widened in surprise. As I envisioned myself embarking on this 3-month grueling regimen, I realized that after the race I would probably not feel much like running anymore.

I admire people who compete in marathons and triathlons. I cheer for them at the finish line. But, the training requirements for these sporting events would quite possibly break me of my "moderate" exercise habit. It took effort to establish low-key, consistent exercise and I do not want to shake that up. I don't want to *begin* an exercise habit again;

keeping an existing habit is far easier. My goal is to be healthy and consistent, not win a race. In terms of extreme exercise, less is more.

I will never discourage anyone from setting a goal to run a marathon. I will, however, recommend people who struggle with maintaining an exercise habit invest in activities they can maintain until they are eighty years old or older. Do things that make you want to get up *the next day* and move again. I politely declined my friend's invitation to run the marathon and volunteered to scream and yell from the sidelines.

Let's not forget about applying this litmus test to what we eat. I don't want to regularly skip breakfast or eat protein bars for lunch until I am eighty. My eating patterns should be sustainable for a good long time, including a healthy breakfast and well-balanced lunch. Happily, this concept of sustainability is really a permission slip to eat wonderful food for the rest of your life because, really, who wants to restrict chocolate? The food we eat for the rest of our lives simply needs to conform to a balanced day. For instance, two chocolate cookies a day will pass the test because they are part of a balanced, sustainable way of life. Two cookies, French fries at lunch, lots of bread, and five handfuls of candy (in addition to full meals) will create imbalance. Over time, this excess will make us fat and, therefore, does not pass the litmus test. Refusing cookies every day is likewise not healthy because denial is unbalanced. Either end of the spectrum—too much or too little—will not build permanently healthy habits.

The Drop

To further illustrate the power of consistent behaviors (over intense short-term diet and exercise programs), consider this object lesson taught by world-class violinist April Moriarty. Try to visualize this: With an eye-dropper squeeze out one drop of water into an extra large, quart-size glass. How much water is in that single drop? Not very much.

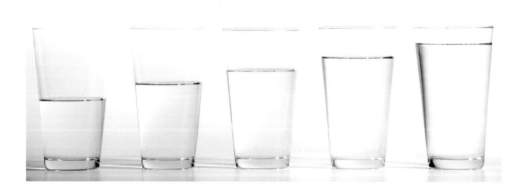

Now, let's say each day of moderate exercise and healthy food equates to one drop of water. As each healthy day passes, you keep squeezing drops of water into your glass. After a month of drops (about 30), you only have about ¼ cup of water in the glass—still not very much. But, here is the magic: if you continue adding a daily drop, you will find after 6 months, your glass is half full. Keep adding one drop a day, and by the end of the year, your glass will be filled to overflowing. Quick, go get another glass.

The power of consistent moderation, applied over a long period of time, produces massive results. Your choice to exercise daily adds drops to your glass. Listening every day to your body and giving it the fuel it needs in the quantity it requires, adds daily drops to your glass. Over a year from now, your glass will run over with drops of water and you will have achieved more than you ever dreamed possible.

Put As Much Energy Into Moderation As Extremes

Why not put as much energy into moderation as extremes? Remember the promises in the introduction of this book: never diet again, never again suffer through roller coaster weight changes, enjoy celebrating the holidays without grieving over how fattening they are, etc.? This is what moderation can do. Moderation can give you the health and beauty you want, while at the same time you live well and abundantly without restriction.

It is tempting to jump on the bandwagon of extreme calorie restriction and intense exercise. If one hour in the gym is great then 2 hours should get me thin in half the time, right? Sorry, this is not exactly the way it works. Consistent moderate activity over time creates a strong, fit body *that stays fit*. When I exert too much, it only makes me sore and exhausted. Excessive workouts require more than twenty-four hours recovery, which makes it more likely I will not return to the gym after my muscles stop hurting. It is far better to exercise consistently at moderate intensity for about 40 minutes, than to go crazy and sweat like a maniac for several hours. Arrange your life to exercise at least five times a week, varying your activity and including stretching and breathing. Moderate intensity means you are breathing deeply, but can still carry on a conversation.

Rest Days

Even moderate exercise requires a periodic rest and recovery day. Tailor your workout schedule around how you feel. Listen to your bones, joints, and muscles for messages of when to rest and which particular exercise to avoid. After three days in a row, I take a day off. This rest day encourages my body to restore and heal. Then I resume exercise for another two days, followed by another day off. An average week contains five exercise days with two days off, spaced when I need it. Read more about muscle recovery in *Should I rest today or am I just being lazy?* in Chapter 7.

Extremes and Metabolism

When I first started becoming healthy, I passed up a litany of tempting extremes such as living on lettuce and tuna fish. Restricting fuel my body needs only slows down my speedy metabolism. But, with a moderate balance of foods, my metabolism starts to work for me. If all required foods are included in a day, I don't feel deprived and, therefore, continue to eat balanced fuel (instead of bingeing on pizza and ice cream).

"*But I want the whole pizza,*" you say? Remember to tune in giving yourself permission to taste and enjoy food. If you remain fully present and taste every single bite, one slice (maybe two) will probably *feel* sufficient. Appropriate portion size is the result of listening to your body and developing a habit of taking "just enough."

Satisfaction also comes from incorporating all the food groups into a meal. A balanced pizza meal would include vegetables and maybe a big green salad. The salad should fulfill over 75% of your total volume of food. Think of splitting your plate in quarters and filling three of those quarters with salad. The fourth quarter is for an appropriate size slice of pizza. It

DAILY FOOD
PROPORTIONS

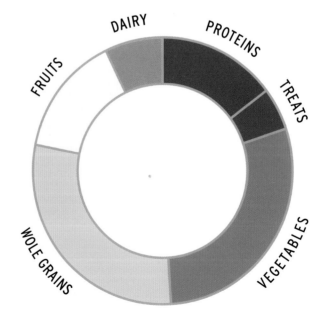

has pepperoni on it? Ok. You want to put creamy dressing on your salad? Ok. Make sure your food tastes worthy of you. It should be delicious enough to savor and, if salad dressing makes that happen, do it. If you balance the pizza with vegetables, it becomes part of a sustainable meal. Now it is time for dessert and you want a little ice cream? Ok. I keep small cups in the house that hold exactly ½ cup. When you want ice cream, use these cups. Eating ½-cup of ice cream will not show up on your thighs. The whole carton…well, I cannot promise anything. The pie chart on the previous page represents general ratios of daily food proportions.

What is Quality Fuel?

What is "quality food?" Based on the above chart, a balanced healthy day would be built on a foundation of whole grains and vegetables, with fruit and proteins augmenting the meal. Dairy, fats, and treats are present, but carefully chosen. Not only is balance achieved with correct proportions, but also with correct timing—giving the body what it needs when it needs it. By way of example, after a good workout I usually need some protein along with whole wheat bread. A turkey sandwich is just the thing. I pile it high with lots of vegetables and some good mustard. A squirt of real mayonnaise finishes it off right. If I need more raw vegetables, I will crunch on a carrot or celery along with my sandwich. I wash it all down with a large tumbler of water. Later in the day, I will have a small treat (something with chocolate) but no more than 3-4 bites—just enough to savor and feel satiated. A sensible dinner and a mug of herb tea at bedtime is the perfect end to a balanced day. If I feel hungry at bedtime, I eat a piece of ripe, seasonal fruit or a piece of whole wheat bread. The last three chapters of this book deal more extensively with what we should eat.

I am often asked for a structured eating plan that details exactly what someone should eat to lose weight. I am reluctant to do this because it prevents people from listening to the needs of *their* body. Instead, they would be following mine. I don't follow a pre-formulated plan every day. I listen to my body and adapt my fuel to the needs of that day. I have, however, outlined some sample days to illustrate better what quality fuel looks like. Please refer to the sample menus on page 155 of the *Reference* section and then talk with, or listen to, your body to create your own balanced diet.

Compensation & Recovery

The key to balancing your diet is to recognize what you already ate. If you had pastry earlier today, you might want to pass on the rolls at dinner. Tomorrow, after a lunch of peanut butter and jelly with pretzels (primarily bread products), at dinner you might want to include a variety of vegetables and lean proteins. It is not necessary to count calories or carbs, just use common sense. Look behind and ahead to build diversity in your diet. Create balance as illustrated in the following sample compensation menus:

SAMPLE COMPENSATION MENUS

	CELEBRATION DAY	DAY AFTER CELEBRATION
Breakfast	Sweet rolls, hot chocolate	Granola and milk, herb tea
Lunch	Ham, potatoes, sour cream, punch, green salad, chips, dip, rolls, jelly	Green salad with beans & almonds, topped with olive oil and lemon juice
Dinner	Ham sandwiches, cheese, white rolls, pasta salad, salted nuts	Vegetable soup with chicken chunks, whole wheat toast
Snack	Pie, ice cream, caramels	Berries

	HEAVY FOOD DAY	COMPENSATION DAY
Breakfast	Eggs and toast	Granola and milk
Lunch	Pasta Alfredo (cream sauce)	Green salad with vegetables
Dinner	Chicken and cheese quesadilla, beans, vegetables, chips, salsa	Fish with brown rice and vegetables
Snack	Chips, cookie, and soda	Fresh fruit and chocolate

After a big holiday feast or big dinner, recover the next day by eating smaller portions and making lean food choices. Think vegetables. When you immediately recover from indulgences, you won't experience weight gain. Avoid bingeing for days on-end because it will start to show. Remember, whatever we regularly do defines us. For instance, if today for lunch you have fried chicken and potatoes, for dinner have green vegetables, whole grains, and a small portion of lean protein. A small portion is between 2-4 ounces (about the size of a deck of playing cards). Remember, most restaurant portions are 2-3 times our needed amount.

Recovery food does not need to be bland. Try sautéed lemon-caper chicken cooked in olive oil and a touch of butter with plenty of vegetables and a side of steamed quinoa. Equally delicious would be oven-roasted fish with broccoli and brown rice. Occasional indulgences like a cream sauce, can be absorbed into your daily lifestyle when you compensate and recover.

As you can tell from this chapter, a holistic approach to food and exercise is key to permanent health. Moderation, consistency, compensation, and recovery are keys to ending dieting as a hobby or obsession. Anything you can do until you are 80 years old is a permanent lifestyle change. Permanent changes produce the results we want—lean, fit, healthy, energetic, active bodies that don't vacillate up and down with the seasons. If health is your lifestyle, no diet is ever needed.

Exercise & Quality Fuel are Partners

Exercise and quality fuel go together like shama lama lama….They are the one-two punches that work and they should not be separated.

There are some very good reasons why some of us cannot exercise. But, there are usually solutions if you are resolved to have activity in your life. If you have a bad leg, swim or exercise in a chair. If you have bad shoulders, ride a stationary bike and walk. If you are not able to exercise at all, breathe deeply using the visualization techniques in Chapter 5. Everyone can find a way to be more active. My 92-year old grandmother tunes in three times a week to her local broadcast of *Sit and Be Fit*. Every Monday, Wednesday, and Friday, from her chair, she elevates her heart rate with upper-body exercises. Do what you can and heed your body's limitations—just get moving.

In order to lose weight, many of us want to forego exercise and focus on restricting calories instead. Don't. Even if you hate exercise, make sure you include both in your healthy lifestyle. Start slow and stay moderate. We were built for motion. The more active we are, the better our marvelous machines work. Sorry to ruin a perfectly good excuse, but unless you are a circus acrobat, normal daily "on the job" activity is generally not enough. Even if it feels like you have walked ten miles at work, get your brow sweaty with regular exercise five times a week.

How do you grow to love exercise? Exercise causes our bodies to release hormones called endorphins. These babies give us a sense of happy exhilaration and well being. They make us feel happy—free of charge. If you haven't experienced your own personal high, you have a real treat coming. In exchange for moderate, pain-free effort, you can have a legal and moral rush every day, in tandem with slimming down to a healthy weight. With exercise we look better, we feel better, and now studies support the fact that exercise helps us manage stress better. The medical world tells us we become smarter when we exercise regularly; we have better recall. Diabetes and hypertension, along with a host of other diseases, are combated directly with exercise and by maintaining a healthy weight. In summary, with exercise we are more beautiful, happier, smarter, calmer, and healthier.

Don't Be Tempted to Lose Weight Too Fast

Let us assume you make a mental shift toward eating healthy and exercising regularly. After a few weeks, you wake up with less excess body fat and a lot more energy. It feels good. But, you still have more weight to lose and you want it off—*now*! So, you find ways to cut more fat or sugar from your diet. Maybe you start skipping meals entirely. You start to ignore hunger pains. You disregard the need for a rest and recovery day and throw in extra workouts to burn a few more calories. Your workouts become longer and harder, making your face turn red, giving you achy muscles, and making you breathe too heavy to talk. This is where I caution people to reign themselves in.

The last thing you want to do is get gung-ho about numbers dropping on a scale. Quick weight loss is the antithesis of permanent weight loss. Perhaps you know this from first-hand experience, which is why you are reading this book. Slow weight loss is fat you never need to lose again. Refer back to Chapters 4 and 5, for more benefits on slow weight loss.

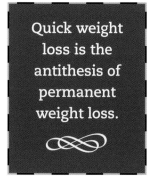

Quick weight loss is the antithesis of permanent weight loss.

As beguiling as it may seem to quickly lose weight, you need to slow it down. The real danger in sudden weight-loss is the tendency to reject the healthy mindset that delivers *permanent* weight control. Notice how quickly we transition from eating healthy to restricting calories outright. Counting calories is not very exciting nor is it particularly useful. It certainly cannot be sustained into old age. And, when pushed too far, exercise can become a calorie-burning means to an end rather than an enjoyable part of an active day—robbing you of joyful movement. A few heart-raising sprints in the middle of a run are part of healthy interval training, but be careful you don't propel your workout to the extreme end of the spectrum and sprint the whole time. You can increase your fitness by picking up the pace and adding intensity while staying within moderate guidelines. Remember to ask yourself: "Can I do this until I am 80?" By paying attention to how you feel, you decide where the line is between moderate and extreme for your own body. It is different for everyone. A moderate spinning class for a 25-year old may be extreme for a 55-year old. On the other hand, a brisk walk with my impressively fast 69-year old aunt is way too fast for me; at 42-years old I have to drop back after a few minutes and go at my own pace which is a little slower. This is ok; my health is not a race.

Ultimately, listen to your body for signals when your exercise is too intense. Listen to your body when it starts to tell you it needs more food and then give it more food. In particular, give your body food it asks for. Sure you may lose weight a bit slower, but you will keep losing until you are at an ideal body size. If slow weight loss helps you become a healthy, strong person, where is the downside? Remember, quick weight loss comes right back and you become the diet industry's favorite customer.

Don't Weigh Yourself Too Often

As you become a regular exerciser, don't become a scale junkie, waking every day to face a number. Weight is just a number. It has nothing to do with how much energy you have or where you are in your pursuit of good health. Besides, numbers on a scale will fluctuate with normal day-to-day activity. You will weigh less in the morning, for instance, than you will each evening. Women may have as much as an eight-pound variance during menstruation. Periods of bloating, holiday-eating, travel food, fasting, and stress will throw the body out of balance. What is the point of weighing ourselves? Unless you suffer from short-term memory loss, you already know whether or not the last three days included great fuel and exercise.

The real danger with stepping on the scale is we tend to have a knee-jerk reaction to the number, whether it is up or down. When the "scale-o-doom" goes up, we tend to restrict food and exercise more intensely or we become frustrated and give up exercise entirely. Even if the scale shows weight loss, we are tempted to think: a little cut back in food worked, a huge cut back in food will *really* speed things up. Notice how we can have the same response whether the scale reveals weight loss or weight gain? Over-intense exercise and calorie restriction (*too much*) are just as non-productive as lack of exercise and overeating (*too little*) because none of these responses boosts your metabolism. If getting on a scale elicits any of these behaviors from you, resist the scale until your weight is no longer an issue.

My yearly doctor's check-up is the only time I get on a scale; even then I cannot be bothered to look at my weight if I happen to be chatting with the nurse. I don't care about the number. I care about how I feel.

If you want to track results, do it with clothing. When clothes fit looser (even after coming out of the wash), you are smaller. But my favorite indicator of weight loss is how I feel during exercise. When I am in balance, my behind doesn't bounce when I run, my abdominal muscles are engaged and firm, my thighs have less thunder, my belly doesn't get in the way when I touch my toes, and my breathing comes easier during household chores. These little markers are better than a scale because they require me to tune in to my body. Remember, your body will tell you what you need, how you are doing, and in what direction you are headed. Trust your body.

Plateaus

When you apply the *Truths* in this book, you may experience weight loss followed by a series of plateaus that make it seem like you are not losing weight. These static periods are merely adjustment phases as our bodies respond in stages. Metabolisms resist change and like to stay consistent, so it can take time for them to shift gears. Your metabolism will accelerate again when it is ready as long as you continue to exercise and eat in balance with your needs. The passage of time will bear this out.

Use this general rule of thumb: it takes three times as long to lose weight as it did to gain it. If you gained ten pounds on vacation last month, anticipate using the next three

TIP 10

Be Patient with Plateaus. It is normal to enjoy quick weight loss at first and then plateau for a while with no visible change. Patiently stay the course. Continue with your healthy behaviors. Over time, your body will get the message that you are a fat-burning machine.

months to restore health and balance to your system—which includes paring off those extra pounds. If you have carried around extra weight for years, allow years to slowly become the optimal size for your particular body.

In Terms of Exercise...

In terms of exercise, what do you have to lose? If after months of exercise you don't lose weight, you still become more cardio-fit and enjoy the happy benefits of activity. But with regular exercise you will loose weight. Next year will come whether you get healthy or not. So, who do you want to be in a year? You might as well become a stronger person with positive habits. Then, as time rolls you down the boulevard of life, you will become a healthier version of yourself.

The salient concept of this chapter is to think permanent, not temporary. Regularly repeated behaviors are the ones that define who we are and how we look. Occasional behaviors have little impact. Over time, new habits become permanent so don't get off track trying to lose weight too quickly with extreme (inherently temporary) programs. The slower we lose, the more our bodies resists gaining it back. We don't want to slow down our metabolism by denying ourselves food. We don't want to be inconsistent with our workouts because it is too hard to start back up again. And, we want to exercise moderately so we feel good enough to do it again tomorrow—enjoying the benefits until we are 80-years old, or older.

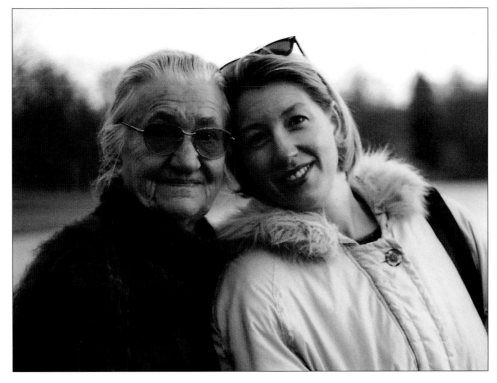

Me with my beautiful 85-year old grandmother. She walked 5 miles a day into her late 80s, and she had fabulous legs!

PHOTO: MARTIN PRIER

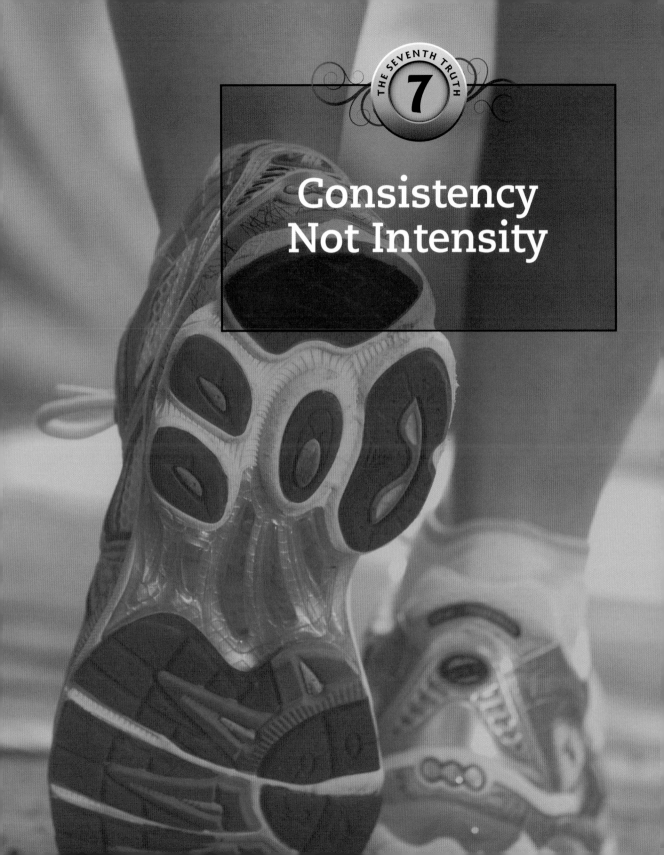

Consistency
Not Intensity

"It happens whether I feel like it or not..."

One morning, a few months into my journey to health, I headed out the door for my daily walk with my baby in the jogging stroller. As we passed my neighbor she said, *"You make me sick, exercising all the time."* She was joking, but her frustration came through the remark. My response came without thinking about it. I said, *"Yup, it happens whether I feel like it or not."* I smiled and went on my way.

Later, at the park, I reflected on this exchange and realized I had made an important discovery. Exercise had become a priority in my life. I did it whether I felt energetic, tired, or busy. In choosing to devote time to my own personal health, I elevated exercise to the same priority as all the other necessary stuff I do in a day, even those things I don't necessarily relish. I don't look forward to doing the dishes, but, because I cannot face the smell of dirty dishes, I load them in the dishwasher and clean out the sink. I don't like paying bills, but I write the checks so my lights don't get turned off. All day long we do things we might not feel inclined to do, but we get them done because we want the results from our efforts. Exercise is important enough to capture a spot on my schedule within moments of waking up or I sometimes set my alarm the night before for an early run. The longer I wait to figure out where it will fit in my day, the less likely I will exercise. It takes a little mental attention to squeeze in exercise, but health is worth the effort.

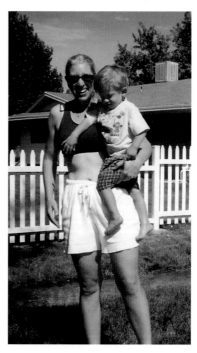

Interestingly, I have seen a positive impact on my family by placing exercise at the top of my daily "to do" list. My teenage daughter views exercise as a normal healthy part of her day. She has a desire to regularly exercise. My two younger boys don't blink an eye when Mom takes time to stretch, breathe, and get moving. The best consequence has been the time I get to spend with my husband and children when they accompany me during a workout. The family is invited whether it is a Latin-rhythm cardio class, a walk on the

A candid shot after a workout, one year after having my second baby.

treadmill, or an hour of volleyball. When I go for a run outside, the little kids ride their bikes until they are big enough to keep up on foot. The babies ride along in the jogging stroller. Sometimes I tell made-up adventure stories to keep our minds occupied. This has become a healthy way to spend quality time together without interruptions. Over the course of those 45-minute exercise sessions, my kids will often share random thoughts with me, things they might be worried about, or things they are excited about that they might not otherwise tell me. Exercising together has sometimes paved the way for important conversations and bonding moments.

Modeling regular exercise for my kids teaches them about a healthy life. It fosters an attitude of respect for Mom because Mom respects herself. They grow up learning healthy behaviors and have a positive attitude about exercise, sports, and activity. They learn how to be fit and healthy. This is a gift to me and to those I love.

The Gift

During live Miracle Pill™ presentations, I like to bring out a nicely wrapped gift box and give it to a random audience member.

I can think of no better way than this object lesson to illustrate the true concept that daily exercise is a gift you give to yourself. Who wouldn't want to receive a valuable gift every day? Who would say, "No thanks, I don't want any desirable stuff today"? Giving yourself the gift of exercise is a validation of your worth. Declare your worth to yourself. It feels good. It makes you happy. It tells the people in your life you have value and deserve all the good moments life has to offer. Regular exercise is an empowering catalyst for change in every aspect of your life. When you make this transition, you know you can do anything.

Reasons to Exercise

Do you need a reason to exercise?
Here are a few key benefits of exercising today:

- Keeps the body moving—because if you don't use it, you lose it!
- Speeds up the metabolism.
- Burns fat.
- Oxygenates the body & brain.
- Improves cognitive functions—studies show exercise makes you smarter (You, the Owner's Manual, by Michael F. Rosen M.D. and Mehmet C. Oz M.D.).

What is Moderate Exercise?

We have talked about the importance of moderate exercise in previous chapters, but because this chapter is all about consistency over intensity, it is vital to define what moderate exercise is and how to achieve it. Moderate exercise feels good and does not hurt. It gets your heart pumping, body sweating, and lungs breathing. If you can carry on a conversation while exercising, your level of intensity is just right. 5-6 times per week of cardio, for 30-50 minutes,

TIP
11

Trick Yourself into Exercise. When I don't feel terribly energetic, I sometimes use a trick to get myself exercising. I simply tell myself to do just 10 minutes of walking. Because 10 minutes is no big deal, I can usually get myself out the door. After walking 10 minutes, I feel warmed up. And, since I am already on the move, I tell myself I will go for a little bit longer—again, no big deal. About 20 minutes into my workout, my endorphins kick in and I start feeling happy. I break into a slow jog, not so much because I need to, but because I want to. As I finish I feel a great sense of satisfaction and accomplishment. I never regret it because I always feel better after exercising than before. Guaranteed!

is plenty—including warm-up and stretching. No need to work out more than once a day. By definition, cardiovascular exercise elevates your heart rate above a normal resting rate for a sustained period of time .

To find your normal resting heart rate, press your finger (not your thumb) under your jawbone on either side of your neck approximately two inches down from your ear. When you find your pulse, count the number of beats in a 10-second period and multiply by six (this will tell you how many beats in a 60 second period). For instance, if you count 11 beats in 10-seconds, multiply 11 x 6 and you get a resting heart rate of 66 beats per minute (bpm).

Now, find your age on the chart on page 82 to determine your target bpm during exercise. This is also your target fat-burning range. For example, at my age (42), I need to raise my heart rate to between 108-135 bpm for 30-50 minutes.

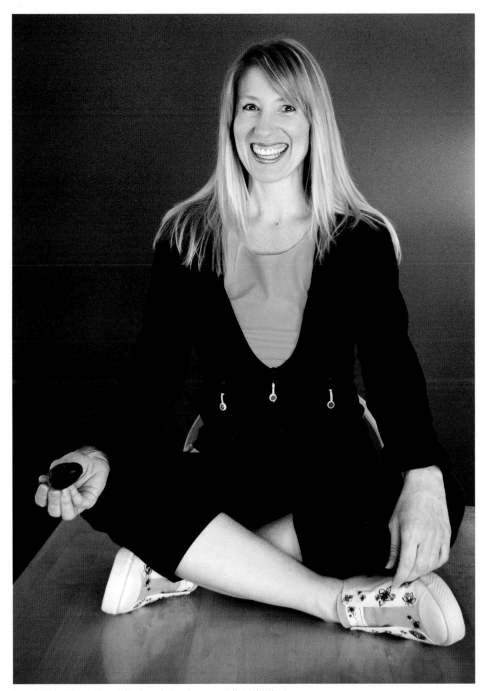

Here I am holding a chocolate-dipped strawberry–call it motivation!

Adult Target Heart-rate Chart										
Age	20 Yrs.	25 yrs	30 yrs	35 yrs	40 yrs	45 yrs	50 yrs	55 yrs	60 yrs	70 yrs
Beats per Minute	120-150	117-146	114-142	111-138	108-135	105-131	102-127	99-120	93-116	90-113

Source: Utah Department of Health, www.hearthighway.org/guidelines

During the first few weeks of exercise, aim for the low end of your target zone—about fifty percent. Check your pulse at least once during exercise, using the above method. Gradually build up to the higher part of your target zone—seventy five percent. The key here is "slowly." For a 20-year old, a bpm of 130 is within the target heart range. For a 70-year old, a bpm of 130 would be too high. If your heart rate goes too high, reduce your intensity to bring it back within range.

Note: A few high blood pressure medications lower the maximum heart rate and thus the target zone rate. If you're taking medicine, ask your physician if you need to use a lower target heart rate.

The figures above are a range, so use them as general guidelines and consult your doctor for your individual target heart rate. Regardless of fitness levels or gender, be aware your maximum heart rate is about 220 minus your age. Do not exceed your maximum heart rate or you will be at risk. Your target heart rate number decreases as you get older, so adjust your goal as time goes on. Other target heart rate charts may have higher numbers if they are designed for more intense interval training. Higher intensity is not necessary. Low-intensity exercise performed consistently is sufficient. You don't need to have a coronary in order to get the job done. Most importantly, listen to your body cues to determine how hard your heart is working and to stay in your target range.

As a suggestion, protect yourself from injury and soreness by using well-fitting shoes appropriate for your activity. Start each workout with at least 10 minutes of walking to warm up. Stretch after a workout instead of before, when your muscles are already warm and are less prone to injury.

Larger Muscle Groups

Have you ever noticed as you repeat any exercise it becomes easier? One reason we sweat less after a month of riding the stationary bike is because we learn to use our muscles more efficiently. This means, with practice, we use less energy to accomplish the same task—which can reduce the metabolic benefit of cardiovascular training. Ideally, we want to speed the metabolism by using all the large muscle groups: thighs, abdominals, back, chest, and shoulder muscles. By varying your activity each day (cross training), you use a variety of large muscle groups, resulting in greater overall fitness.

Cross training also minimizes stress on any single area of the body while it improves coordination and balance. Distributing the work between many muscle groups prevents injury due to over-repetition of one particular movement. Additionally, it keeps you from getting bored of your exercise routine. Your soul stays inspired as your body enjoys the benefits of varying kinds of motion.

Choose the aerobic activities you can enjoy with regularity: swimming, dancing, tennis, walking, yoga, etc. Throw in new activities to broaden your regimen: skating, basketball, jogging, hiking, weight training, martial arts, volleyball, golf, etc. If life gives you an opportunity to move your glorious body, take it.

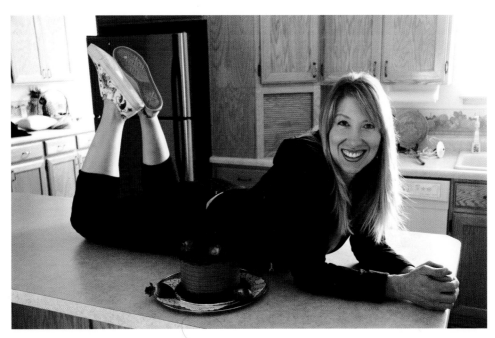

Exercise has its benefits...namely, chocolate cake!

Getting Going

Game Plan for Non-exercisers

If you haven't exercised for a while (or ever) start small and easy. Begin with 5-10 minutes of moderately paced walking, followed by easy stretching and deep breathing. Can you find time for 5-10 minutes of "you time" in your day? Really, this is all it takes to begin a lifelong exercise program.

After a week, increase your activity to 15-20 minutes. Incorporate resistance training with light weights (between 1-3 pounds) and a few repetitions (maybe 8-10 reps). For instance, by the second week, you might be walking 15 minutes, doing 8 modified push-ups, 20 abdominal crunches, one set of 10 bicep curls using handheld weights, and 10 lunges. Following this, you might stretch for another 5 minutes, using deep breaths and slow, sustained exhales. Over the following months, build up weight training to include multiple sets. Use correct techniques to protect your body. If you need advice on proper form, consult a good exercise manual or a personal trainer. Even better, ask a friend with exercise experience to evaluate your form and make suggestions.

See how nice it is to embrace moderation? There is nothing painful or complicated about starting to exercise. By your third week, increase your intensity bit by bit. For instance, if you enjoy walking, increase your pace to a brisk walk, swing your arms as you walk to pump up your heart rate, and contract your abdominal muscles for 30-second intervals.

If your exercise of choice is swimming, start gently and gradually increase your duration and intensity. Work to kick your legs a little harder during the second week. If you decide to use an aerobic video, increase your intensity slightly after a few weeks. For maximum fun, do a different activity every day or rotate exercises you enjoy. You might dance one day, jog the next, and practice yoga after that. Just remember to start slow and easy, building your duration up over time.

TIP 12

Don't Push Too Hard. It is a natural inclination to exercise harder then we should. Resist the urge. Better to feel like you are not exercising hard enough, and to keep doing it, than to overexert and break your habit because of pain or fatigue. The habit is more valuable than the extra calories you may have burned. Why? Because, we want a lifetime of sleek muscles, instead of just one weekend in skinny jeans.

Game Plan for Exercisers

If you are already in the habit of exercising, don't launch into your first week with an hour of cardiovascular exercise. Instead, re-set your metabolism with only 20 minutes of daily exercise followed by easy stretches. I know you can do more—but don't. Slowly build up to a longer workout. This process of implementing moderation is part of changing the way you think. It is important to train your mind and body in the habit of consistent moderation, instead of frequent extremes. You may find exercising 20 minutes, 5 times a week, is considerably less activity than you are accustomed to. That's ok. Do a little less for the first 2 weeks. Allow your body to benefit from consistency instead of intensity.

If you are a tri-athlete who cannot maintain a healthy weight without several hours of exercise every day, set your timer and force yourself to stop after 20 minutes—and allow yourself two weeks to build up to 40 minutes. After a few months of 40-50 minute workouts, your body will learn to burn fat for fuel from the demands of regular moderate exercise. "A few months?" you ask. Don't panic. You are trying to re-set your body so it can accomplish health and wellness with *sustainable* efforts. Several hours of punishing exercise every day will eventually lead to injury and a worn-out attitude. It cannot be maintained into old age. However, 40 minutes of moderate exercise, followed by stretching, can be maintained. Go for the minimum, but do it regularly.

Life Outside the Gym

When I first started my health program, I did what most of us do—I went to the gym. I was considerably larger than the other patrons, and on my second day, I went to get a drink at the drinking fountain. A man came up behind me to get in line but he awkwardly hung back, taking his spot only after a thinner woman got in line behind me. He could not even bear to *stand in line* behind a "fat girl." Abashed, I looked down at my feet to spare him the trauma of direct eye contact. Could fat be contagious? Would my bending over to take a drink overwhelm his delicate sensibilities? From his averted eyes and disgusted expression, there could be no doubt for the motives behind his bizarre behavior.

TIP 13

No Shame. Do not ever allow embarrassment, shame, pride, humiliation, or any other excuse to keep you from kindly taking care of your body. In the words of Eleanor Roosevelt, "No one can make you feel inadequate without your consent."

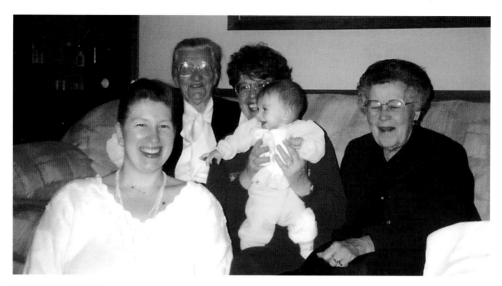

Above: Me around the time of the "gym incident." This photo includes four generations of beautiful women—including both of my pretty grandmothers, my lovely Mom and adorable daughter.

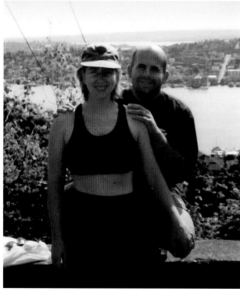

Left: Here I am in Seattle with my husband Jon, 3 years after the "gym incident."

Clearly, the gym was not right for me. Those kinds of situations were not what I needed at that point in my transition. I wanted to feel good about myself—at every stage of fitness. I promptly found a park near my house with a walking path, and I purchased inexpensive exercise videos to do at home on rainy days. Rather than dwell on the injustice and humiliation of my public spandex moment, I kept my eye on the ball and developed a strategy for success.

Should I rest today or am I just being lazy?

There is a difference between needing a day off from exercise and just being lazy. Get to know the difference. Some days you may feel sluggish. The best remedy for feeling like you have anvils in your hip pockets is exercise. Power through the doldrums and enjoy the invigorated high you get from exercise. However, there will be lethargic days when you may be fighting illness or injury. You may be seriously in need of sleep. Perhaps you are achy from a previous activity. Decide whether or not to exercise based on the messages your body sends you. There is a thin line between working out with a mild case of the sniffles (which sometimes makes you feel better) and depleting your immunities with strident exercise to the point that your symptoms present more severely. When you need to take a recovery day, take it—or pay the price. Only by listening to your body will you know when you should reserve your strength and postpone today's exercise or when you should rock-on and workout.

As we age, we need more time for recovery. After lifting boxes into storage, playing a recreational game of touch football, or throwing a wedding for your daughter, you may need an extra recovery day. As a teenager, I pulled all-nighters and still went to the gym at 6:00 a.m. the next morning. I don't do that anymore. The point is to listen to your body as you get older. If you ignore the need for rest, you may get sick or injured—which may interrupt your consistent exercise program.

There are times when we have no choice but to postpone our exercise program for an extended period of time. Sometimes life demands that we take care of a sick loved one, undergo surgery, cope with death, trauma, or travel. When interruptions happen, keep your thoughts on track with healthy eating. Squeeze in exercise when you can, and then ease back into your regular routine as soon as possible, without overexerting.

Body Conversations

As you exercise and eat, have a body conversation. This is a fun activity because at any age you can be delightfully surprised at the many messages you will receive from your body. Set a watch or timer if you need to.

During Exercise

- Notice how you feel 5 minutes into your exercise warm up.

- Notice how you feel 10 minutes into your cardiovascular exercise (this is the part of your workout that gets you breathing heavier and makes your heart beat faster).

- Notice how long it takes to get an endorphin high. In other words, how long into your workout does it take to feel happy? When your body releases endorphins, you might get a burst of energy or feel like singing. You might have clarity of thought or even a stream of ideas. It might take consistent exercise (2-3 weeks) before your brain produces noticeable levels of endorphins. Keep exercising consistently to receive this chemical benefit. It is free, morally acceptable, and not fattening. Pretty groovy! See Tip #9 on page 72.

⚒ Notice how your body feels when you exercise too strenuously.

While Eating

⚒ Notice how your body and mind feel 30 minutes after eating what your body asked for. You should feel light and energized—ready to move. You will not feel bloated and stuffed.

⚒ Pay attention to how food tastes when you choose exactly what your body needs. For instance, on a day when you need greens, choose a fresh spinach salad with chicken (instead of pork ribs). How does it taste? Do you feel satisfied?

⚒ Notice how you feel 2 hours *after* fulfilling your body's need for healthy fuel. Because you listened to your body at dinner, your metabolism may speed up and you might be hungry. For a snack try a piece of seasonal fruit and plenty of water. If you ever feel shaky, eat something. Try to include low-fat protein in your snack menu to prevent this feeling (like a handful of nuts). I enjoy a rolled-up slice of deli turkey stuffed with a pear slice and celery spear. Sliced chicken or boiled egg with cucumber spears and bleu cheese dressing are another favorite.

⚒ Notice how your body feels after eating cheese fries with dipping sauce (or your gut-buster of choice). Learn which foods stimulate your desire for movement and which ones slow you down. For instance, after eating sushi and miso soup, I feel like running a race. After a steak and a stuffed potato, I feel like taking a nap.

TIP 14

Use the Time You Have. Even if you only have 10 minutes today, use that precious time to exercise because doing so maintains your exercise habit.

Caution for Extreme Exercisers

We all know why we don't exercise, but why do some of us over-exercise? Many are addicted to the high of exercise, while others fuel a sense of control through grueling physical challenges. Some extreme exercisers do it so they can eat those extra calories without getting fat. Problems arise if this kind of abuse goes on too long—namely, when the workouts stop, we pack on the pounds because our food choices are incongruent with our calorie expenditures—while at the same time our metabolisms decrease. If you find yourself falling into this category, decrease your intensity and amount of exercise. Reduce your food intake commensurate with your new—moderate—workouts. This does not need to take the form of restriction or denial. Listen to your body cues about food choices, portion sizes, and meal timing. You may need to rethink habits and pare down to a simpler diet of unprocessed food (think fresh fruit and vegetables, whole grains, lean proteins, and very little drive-thru). If you find you are not hungry at the usual time, wait to eat until you are.

Equity between calories consumed and calories burned reinforces a fast metabolism and keeps you from gaining weight. If you have been ignoring your body's signals for a long time with far too much intensity and by giving it too much (and possibly the wrong kinds of) fuel, it may take weeks for your body to start signaling its needs. Use patience until you start hearing the messages your body will send you. While you wait, use common sense. Choose unprocessed, healthy food. Have a small treat every day without any guilt. Fully taste your food so you feel satisfied afterward.

What About Those Who Need a Big Push?

We are conditioned to believe it takes a lot of gearing up to start an exercise program. I hope the previous paragraphs have set your mind at ease and convinced you to merely put one drop in the exercise bucket each day. However, there are some of us that need to be shot with a stun gun just to get off the couch. If this is you, I confess the best out-of-the-gate motivator for me has always been food. In this instance, use your desire for food to your advantage: select an amazing treat every day and *earn it* with exercise. Remember to schedule your exercise first thing each day so it doesn't get swept under the carpet of your busy life. Make your sweat happen and then reward yourself with a treat. Listen to your body to know when to eat the treat and how much your body wants. Taste it. No guilt.

Something magical happens when exercise becomes a habit. Over time, the former incentive of food becomes less important because exercise is its own reward—namely, it makes you feel good and look good. But, for now, just enjoy looking forward to a brownie with nuts and go put on your running shoes.

Exercise Nuts & Bolts. *Choose exercise that increases respiration to a deep, yet comfortable level. Take weeks, if you need, to build up to 30-50 minutes. Exercise should not be painful—ever! Your breathing should be deep but not leave you gasping or lightheaded. You will know you are at the correct level of intensity if you are able to talk throughout the activity. Maintain enough intensity to challenge your body, but moderate enough to feel like exercising the next day. Sustain your duration long enough to fully use your muscles, but not so long you feel drained and sore. One-size-fits-all rules do not apply to you. Just as you listen to your body with regards to food, also listen as you exercise to learn what your parameters should be.*

Rhetorical Exercise Q&A

Question: Does the thought of intense workouts six days a week for the rest of your life seem overwhelming?

Answer: It should. Painful and obsessive intensity is not a part of a healthy, moderate lifestyle. No wonder some of us procrastinate exercise for another day—the prospect of self-punishment is daunting and no fun at all. However, if you take the pain and intensity out of the exercise equation, you are left with all the benefits of exercise and none of the drawbacks. *Change your task from intense exercise to moderate consistency, and you change your whole attitude.*

Question: Could you enjoy a 25-minute walk with a few stretches at the end?

Your Answer: _____

_____

Question: After a few months of walking, could you add 5-10 minutes of slow jogging into the middle of your walk?

Your Answer: _____

_____

Question: Does stretching and breathing at the end of your walk feel good?

Your Answer: _____

_____

The Power of Today

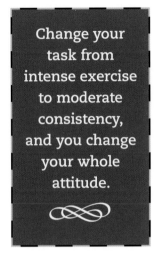

Change your task from intense exercise to moderate consistency, and you change your whole attitude.

Consistency is really about moderation and moderation means living well, one-day-at-a-time. This one-day-at-a-time *truth* is important. Instead of gearing up to start a new diet or exercise program that you will need to maintain for several months (or else you will feel like a loser), try limiting your focus to today. Just take care of today. Listen, eat, enjoy, exercise, breathe, and be kind to yourself—today! These are the only requirements on your plate. We don't have a guarantee on tomorrow. So, let's not worry about tomorrow or get overwhelmed with future responsibilities. Your only real power is in today's choices. The greatest achievers in history understood this principle. Nothing is accomplished without completing today's required work.

Yesterday is history. Don't beat yourself up over last night's cheesecake. It is old news—gone and digested. No one on earth can change yesterday. But, today I can listen to my body and allocate 30-50 minutes for gentle exercise. I can go to bed a little earlier. Why? Because getting to bed earlier helps me get up earlier which opens an exercise window in tomorrow (See *Tip #19* in Chapter 9). But don't get bent out of shape about tomorrow. We only need to focus on bedtime today. Just enjoy today. Doesn't it take the pressure off to approach each day as a complete unit—start to finish? Fill today with good choices and then decide again tomorrow to make more healthy choices.

Imagine each day as a perfect circle, containing all you need within it. Each circle is complete and stands alone. Simply fill each circle (day) with your needs. See Chapter 10 for a graphic of the entire spectrum of foods to be consumed in a day. This paradigm of living each day one-at-a-time, for its greatest benefit, applies to nutrition, exercise, and any other endeavor you choose.

That's it. Nowhere are you committing to a 2-hour kick-boxing class that makes you feel like you are going to have a heart attack. What a relief.

However, should you decide to take a class, take a break if your heart rate gets too high. Get a drink. If you have fulfilled your 40 minutes (or however long your body tells you to go), stop and stretch. Avoid comparisons with the über kick-boxers and don't make it a competition. You are there to fulfill today's health as part of your regular, daily routine. Don't blow it for tomorrow by trying to "out kick" everyone in the class.

Tricks For a Stronger Core

To augment your cross training, here are tricks to strengthen your core muscles (your abdominal and back muscles) while going about your everyday activities:

Engage abdominal muscles—

✻ When exercising—use your abs to do push-ups or to finish your run.

✻ When bending over—contract your core muscles to prevent back strain.

✻ When tired—use your center to sit up straight, to refresh the body and align the spine.

✻ When doing household chores—reach and bend with a tight tummy.

✻ When driving—contract upper, middle, and lower abdominal muscles at every stoplight. Hold for 30-second intervals. Try this on airplanes too.

✻ Before lifting heavy objects—engage core muscles, bend knees and lift with legs.

✻ To correct posture—flex your abs as you straighten spine and pull back shoulders. You will notice immediate posture improvement.

Resistance Training

Resistance training (using weights for resistance) strengthens joints and muscles while increasing bone density. We know pushing, pulling, and lifting are necessary for long-term health. When performed at least three times per week, strength training can build better bone health and connective tissue, tone muscles, burns fat so your muscles are leaner, increases joint health, reduces stress and anxiety, develops balance, increases range of motion, prevents injury, strengthens heart and lungs, and increases energy. One of the biggest benefits is the increase to your metabolism.

Heavy weights are not required. Rather, use light-to-moderate weights and complete a couple of sets of 10-20 repetitions. No need for fancy equipment either. Simple hand weights and calisthenics will do. To use your own body weight to create resistance, try doing forward lunges. Make sure your forward foot lands heal-to-toe and your front knee does not exceed a 90-degree angle. As few as 8 repetitions on each side will get you breathing. Consult a personal trainer or an exercise manual for examples of this and other exercises. An internet search on "resistance training" will provide you with endless results. Use reliable information and common sense.

Ten modified push-ups will give you all the benefits just mentioned above. "Modified" means your upper body performs a standard push up while your lower body rests on the floor on the tissue above your knees (not your kneecaps) instead of your feet. Keep your abdominal muscles engaged and your body flat like a table; don't stick your fanny in the air.

Try doing two sets of 10 squats with your feet hip distance apart. Keep your weight on your heels, arms forward, and tighten your legs and buttocks as you straighten up into a standing position. If you need to do fewer reps today than you did last week, heed those body prompts. I recommend doing some form of aerobic activity first and then resistance training while your muscles and lungs are warmed up. Finish with stretching and breathing for an invigorated body. In addition to lunges, push-ups, and squats, there are hundreds of simple at-home exercises you can incorporate into your week. If an exercise feels painful or risky, don't do it.

Here is a look at a week's worth of moderate, consistent exercise:

Weekly Exercise Components

Aerobic Exercise

4-6 times per week of aerobic exercise, for 30-50 minutes (including warm up), low intensity

- Engage in cardiovascular activities of your choice
- Before commencing, warm up slowly with walking and light, easy movement
- Cross-train
- Pay attention to how you feel at 10 minutes, 30 minutes, etc…
- Oxygenate

Stretching & Breathing

4–6 times per week after your cardiovascular workout, for 5–10 minutes

- Stretch when muscles are warm
- Use yoga breathing (see following section)
- Visualize
- Realign posture
- Lengthen muscles

Resistance Training (Hand Weights & Body Weight)

3 times per week, for 10-20 minutes

- After aerobic exercise
- Work upper body with weights—bicep curls, tricep curls, etc.
- Modified push ups
- Tricep dips
- Squats & legs
- Abdominals

Yoga Breathing

Use Yoga Breathing During Exercise and While Stretching

Yoga breathing is the intake and exhalation of the breath at strategic moments. It teaches you to manipulate breath for increased strength, flexibility, and relaxation. To get the most out of your workout, employ the following yoga breathing techniques: After warming up with any aerobic activity, take several deep breaths through your nose and exhale completely through your mouth. Breathe normally for a minute and then do it again, picturing the air rushing into your body as colored vapor rushing to the ends of your extremities—all the way from to your hair to your toes. Don't overdo it or you will get lightheaded. Visualize your body in the ideal form you would like it to be (see Chapter 5 for more on visualization). Celebrate your glorious body. Notice how you feel after breathing this way.

Try yoga breathing while stretching, inhaling through your nose as you settle into a position. Exhale while you go deeper into the pose. Inhale again to release a pose and transition to a new stretch. Keep your breathing steady and don't hold your breath. For a more advanced form of breathing refer to the *Breathing Technique* section in Chapter 2.

I recommend deep breathing several times throughout your day. It reduces stress and keeps your metabolism humming along. Oxygenation is so effective that you will see immediate increases in your metabolic machine, encouraging it to burn fat for fuel.

Use Yoga Breathing After Stretching

After you stretch, sit quietly or lie down for a few moments to pay attention to your breath. Slow your breathing. Relax your body from your head to your toes. Calm your mind. Ask yourself how you feel. You should feel relaxed and energized. As you do this short relaxation technique, allow your breath to become quiet and shallow. The stillness of your body allows you to notice your corporeal self in a way you could not during the hustle and bustle of your daily routine.

To learn more about yoga and breathing techniques, take a yoga class or rent a good DVD (I recommend *Kathy Smith's New Yoga Workout©*). Generalize yoga breathing techniques into other activities as part of your daily stress management. Inhale when you reach up to grab hold of a heavy object, like the ladder in the garage. Exhale to lower it back down. When you pick up the bag of groceries, contract your abs and inhale, slowly exhaling as you set it down on the counter. Inhale to lean over and plug in your printer. Exhale as you push the cord into the plug, then inhale to move your body back into an upright position. As you pay your bills, keep your breathing steady (sometimes this is hard to do!).

Yoga breathing is not only for meditative types. Increasing the circulation of oxygen to our blood makes sense. Here is a short list of the benefits of deep breathing:

- Helps prevent muscle soreness
- Oxygenates muscles, organs, and your brain—Yup, it makes you smarter!
- Sends blood through the body which carries away toxins
- Increases flexibility if used in combination with stretching
- Makes us feel energized and relaxed

Your Exercise Plan

Create your own exercise plan and make any changes to the following three statements to suit your body.

1 I want to raise my heart rate to a fat-burning level. I will do it _____ times per week. Here's how: _____

_____

_____

_____

_____

_____

_____

_____

2 I want to build lean muscle mass with resistance training. I will do it _____ times per week. Here's how: : _____

_____

_____

_____

_____

_____

_____

3 I want to increase flexibility, strength, and oxygenation with slow stretching. I will do this _____ times per week. Here's how: _____

_____

_____

_____

_____

_____

_____

_____

Other goals:

4 _____

_____

_____

_____

_____

_____

5 _____

_____

_____

_____

_____

_____

_____

_____

6 _____

_____

_____

_____

_____

_____

_____

_____

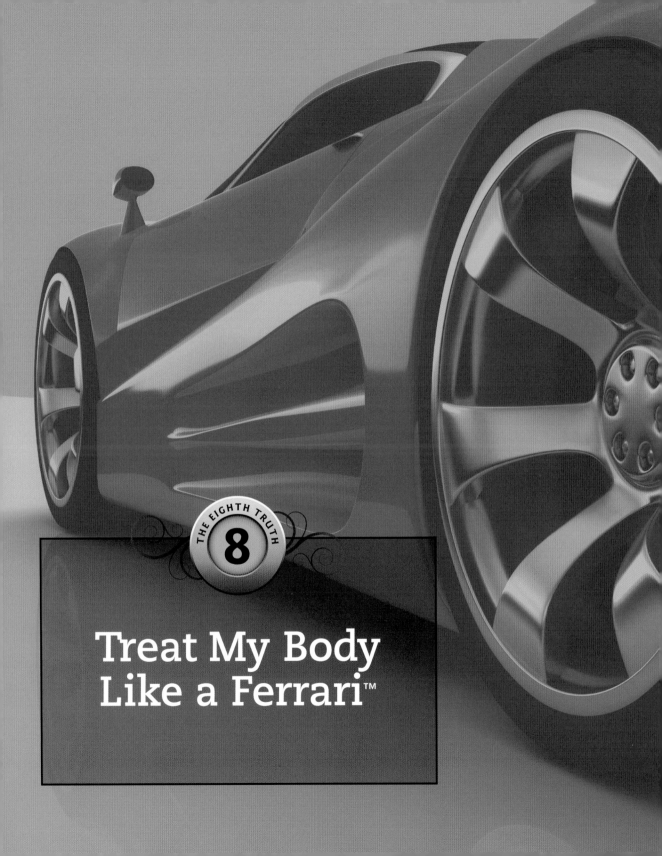

Treat My Body Like a Ferrari™

Like any finely-tuned machine, we must care for our bodies with special attention. High-grade fuel, maintenance, and regular exercise keep the equipment running at optimal performance. The manner in which you see your body dictates how you treat it. If you believe you have a sleek sports car under the hood, you will maintain it as such. On the other hand, if you cultivate a clunker with neglect and poor fuel, you will get no better than a clunker. The following chapter explores ways to boost the performance of your engine and transform yourself into a high-performance machine.

Food Serves Two Purposes—Fuel & Pleasure

Healthy eating fulfills only two purposes: fuel and pleasure. Any other reason for eating creates problems and leads to imbalance.

Let's talk about embracing pleasure. Eating is meant to be a pleasurable activity. Diet programs, overly thin celebrities, and our "wacked-out" culture combine to discourage the enjoyment of food, as if we are somehow weak for succumbing to the delights of eating.

> **Take time to savor the flavor instead of stuffing the mouth and headin' south.**

But the truth is we are designed to smack our lips and declare "*yum!*" It does not seem reasonable to disregard our visceral responses to delicious food. Are we supposed to engage superhuman discipline and ignore the enticements of instinctive pleasure? How very puritan. You can't fight nature, baby—and why would you? Personally, I could use a bit more pleasure in my day and, therefore, will embrace any opportunity to enjoy pleasure—sans guilt.

Say yes to the pleasure of eating and you essentially give yourself permission to taste food. In *Tip #1*, at the beginning of this book, I encouraged you to tune in to your food. Only then can you focus your attention on taste and the sublime pleasure of good food. In this way, you will also hear prompts of satisfaction and completion when you have had enough. For instance, take the dinner roll, put it on a plate, slather it with butter, and eat one bite at a time, allowing the full impact of the taste to hit your brain. Continue to enjoy while assessing the taste. Stop when your attention is directed elsewhere. Take time to savor the flavor instead of "stuffing the mouth and headin' south."

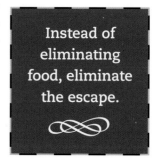

> **Instead of eliminating food, eliminate the escape.**

During a meal, when you begin to emotionally withdraw, force yourself to stay in the present, focused on your food. Be kind to yourself and give your body a pass on the self-punishment. Eat and stay engaged with the people around you, allowing only a grateful enjoyment of pleasure to exist. As you require yourself to resist using food as an emotional escape, over time this new behavior will become the norm and you will reduce cravings and binges, enjoy portion control, and deactivate eating triggers. Unhealthy habits can only exist when you willingly use food as an escape. Instead of eliminating food, eliminate the escape. This way you can have your cake and eat it, too!

Ways to Experience Pleasure

- Put food on a plate and sit down.

- Try to enjoy peaceful conversation during mealtimes.

- Don't sneak food in by eating alone, eating fast, or while doing other things (that's not pleasure—that is escape). Escapism is the root of binge eating.

- Own your food choices. Make it a conscious decision. Choose pleasure *not* restriction. Denial only makes us want something more. Say out loud, *"Yes, I will have one cupcake."*

- If "just one" is never enough, give yourself permission to enjoy an appropriate amount and truly taste, enjoying that portion.

- Treats are normal and healthy. Don't beat yourself up over a small portion of something yummy. Avoid going down the road of self-punishment that may lead to bingeing.

- Rather than feel deprived that a portion size is not big, enjoy the anticipation of tasting with all your senses and the satisfaction that comes after. *Quality* makes us full and happy—not quantity.

- Ask your body if you *need* a treat. You might be surprised when one day you do and another day you do not.

Escape Is a Six-Letter Word

Because we are discussing escape, let's put it under the microscope and find some truth about this misunderstood concept. Escaping is not inherently bad or good. Escapes can be healthy or destructive, depending on how they affect your life. Reading an inspiring book is an escape, as is taking a tennis lesson, shoe shopping, and test-driving a BMW™. But when an escape has a negative impact on your life, it is destructive and needs to be replaced. Too much shoe shopping with a credit card cannot end well. Smoking is another example of a bad escape. Eating a bowl of ice cream every night before bed, while surfing the web, is also a destructive escape.

On the flip side, healthy activities can become unhealthy escapes as well, if they are taken to the extreme. For instance, if you stay up all night to read that inspiring book, the next day you are going be tired. If you do it night after night, that habit will eventually get in the way of your work responsibilities. Something as innocuous as a ballroom dance class has the potential to turn into an unhealthy habit. Let us suppose you attend a dance class and find yourself intensely attracted to another student—who happens to be married. Now you have a fascination you don't want to quit—that carries a load of potential problems. Be aware, escapes can be either healthy or unhealthy and, as time goes on, they may develop unexpected consequences.

Having said all that, in terms of food, escape is *never* a good idea.

TIP 16

Distractions While Eating. While you establish new habits, avoid watching television or reading while you eat. Eliminate distractions so you can taste your food. Frequently, we zone out as we eat and find we ate more than we wanted or needed because we were distracted. Later, after you have established a new habit of consuming only what it takes to become satisfied, you will be able to eat popcorn during a movie or have a bowl of chili during the big game and still hear your body's signals.

Lose the Guilt

Discard unnecessary guilt. Little girls and boys are bullied and called names when they show even the smallest amount of fat. From a very young age, we have learned to revile extra weight and embrace the notion we are bad for having it. Thin is admirable, fat is repellent. "Fat guilt" is a huge part of our collective psyche. While fat is certainly not something to which we should aspire, it is not a singular indicator of a "bad" person. There is no natural correlation between "fat'" and "bad." Yet, the guilt goes on.

One kind of useless guilt is the "post-meal" kind. We are conditioned to self-punish for enjoying Thanksgiving dinner, pie and all. We tend to look back on a great meal with equal parts delight and regret. Have you ever gotten up from the table and yearned to unbutton your pants, hating yourself for overindulging? Sure it's not your most shining moment, but a day or two of recovery eating is all it takes to negate any damage done; so, why the self-hate?

We should enjoy Thanksgiving dinner. The desire for pleasure is natural and normal. Guilt for enjoyment of food is the poor country cousin to obsessing over body flaws—I've got varicose veins, my butt is too big, my doo-dads are too small—that kind of obsessing. Reproach for imperfections is reinforced in every medium, at every age, and on every social level. We feel discontent because our body doesn't look quite like an arbitrary standard that was, incidentally, photo-shopped for the cover of a magazine. Lose the guilt for enjoying food and, in doing so, you will more readily embrace your body as a uniquely designed machine—shaped for your journey in this life.

If you get out of balance and stop listening to your body's cues, cut yourself some slack and assess your life. Have you been stressed, sick, traveling, recently divorced, pregnant, medicated, or have you experienced any of the myriad of factors that take us away from a balanced routine? Life is unpredictable. Sometimes, we don't have control over our menu choices or the quantity of food we eat. There are critical business dinners that wind on course after course and, sometimes, you need to grease the wheels to ink the deal. The last dinner I had with my German Grandmother before she died involved three pieces of apple cake. I flew 2000 miles to see her, she baked it, and, by golly, when she insisted I have a third piece, I said thank you and enjoyed that cake with gusto. Later that day I walked several miles and ate salad, but I don't regret the sweet memory of that apple cake.

The point is there are times when we don't have control over all aspects of life and we need to accept them as such—without guilt. Skip the "I don't have any self control" drama. Rather than beat yourself up, just resume listening with self-respect and have a recovery day.

My Triggers

Allowing pleasure to return to your meals helps eliminate cravings and binges, but we all have certain triggers that make us want to eat compulsively. Know your automatic eating triggers and diffuse them with balanced attitudes toward food. The following are my eating triggers. Most of them don't affect me anymore, but some still itch at the back of my mind.

1   Mom's refrigerator door

2   Arguments with my husband

3   Loneliness

4   Boring social events

5   Anxiety over money or personal relationships

6   Stress from too little "me" time

7   Avoidance when I don't want to hear bad news

8 Denial—when I stuff truth by stuffing my mouth

9 Anger—because it is easier to punish myself with a binge than to get angry and face the consequences

10 Escape from reality

11 Pity party—"What did I do to deserve this…"

12 Need for control—overeating provides a false sense of control as it creates the illusion of taking action

What are Your Eating Triggers?

These are the things that make you want to mistreat your body. Over the next few pages, you will have the opportunity to identify your compulsive behaviors caused by these triggers. For now, just focus on your triggers. List the top ten below.

1 _____

2 _____

3 _____

4 _____

5 _____

6 _____

7 _____

8 _____

9 _____

10 _____

Now, put a check mark by your 3 main eating triggers—the ones you encounter most. These three triggers can be eliminated first by simply tasting your food and giving yourself permission to completely enjoy it. If your trigger is the smell of fast food and pulling through the drive thru is your compulsion, make a point to sit quietly with your hamburger and French fries, tasting each and every bite. Is the hamburger bun overly soft and soggy? Are the fries limp and greasy? Is there enough flavor on the burger to justify the massive amount of fat contained between the bun? What is the dominant flavor, salt? Even if every aspect of that burger and fries is perfect in its preparation and tastes sublime, it is the conscious act of tasting that helps take the energy out of compulsions. Notice how quickly you can deflate these triggers with your newfound approach of recognizing them as triggers, tuning in when you eat, and losing the guilt. Continue to de-activate all of your triggers.

Compulsions

What is a compulsion? To effectively discuss this topic, let's define compulsion as responding to our triggers over and over, despite unwanted consequences. Seemingly, we cannot stop ourselves. As you practice the concepts in this book and learn how to redirect behaviors toward more desirable outcomes, there are three cautions you should be aware of. First, prevent the spread of compulsions from one area of your life to another—because, like a virus, they ooze into unwanted places. For instance, it is easy to generalize my compulsive act of opening Mom's refrigerator door within minutes of arriving at her house to opening my own fridge every time I get home. Additionally, if I reach for chocolate whenever I hear bad news in a telephone conversation, I need to be careful not to generalize the use of chocolate to cope with stressful face-to-face conversations. Limiting compulsions to their narrow origin is the first step toward mastering them.

Second, take care compulsions do not become habits even after the trigger has passed. For instance, in a stressful work situation, we might start spending more time with muffins and soda in the break room. Soon, muffins and soda become important—needed. But even after things calm down at work, we may still seek out the break room and feel a compulsive need for muffins and soda. By way of another example, a bag of licorice might become the comfort for someone caring for an elderly parent and that bag of licorice can quickly become a regular part of each day. However, when the situation changes and the caregiver is relieved of their responsibilities, the licorice might remain a daily habit. Over time, a behavior that started out as a temporary compulsion can become a habit—like muffins, soda, and licorice. Even if we no longer remember why we needed them, we still want them because they are now habits.

Thirdly, compulsions can become dangerous and may require professional help. I am referring to diseases like anorexia and bulimia. They stem from control issues and feed on compulsive behaviors. Unchecked, these self-abuses can result in death. In conjunction with these diseases, I cannot overly caution against the misuse of diet pills, energy stimulants (caffeine drinks), and laxatives as well as a litany of other addictions. If you experience symptoms of anorexia or bulimia, or even dabble in these dangerous behaviors, please contact a doctor immediately and get help.

Replace Compulsions

To overcome compulsions, don't try to eliminate them—replace them. Studies suggest we overcome compulsive behaviors better when we replace them with a healthier action, than when we try to stop them outright. So, now that you have listed your triggers, use the chart below to identify your compulsions and choose a corresponding replacement behavior. Just to be clear, compulsions are different from triggers—they are the *response* to your triggers listed above. For instance, my trigger is my Mom's refrigerator door and my compulsion is to open that door. As a replacement, I now ask for a hug. She loves to give me hugs, I love to receive them—it works out nicely. When I receive a stressful telephone call, instead of chomping down chocolate, I think, *"It will all work out. Breathe. You don't have to come up with a solution to everything right this second."* I digest this new monologue—instead of fats and carbohydrates. The person on the phone deserves the full me, not a diluted version who has momentarily escaped on the Hershey™ highway.

You don't have to know why you have a compulsion in order to replace it. Often, the replacement act will reveal the "why." Instead of toiling through years of therapy to figure out the cause, decide today to replace your compulsion with a positive substitute. (Therapy is a helpful and often necessary treatment for mental illness, but it may be superfluous in some cases when compulsions merely require a replacement substitute.) Take action. Even if you never discover the root of the compulsion, it will not matter because if you exchange it out for a healthy habit it will no longer plague your life. In my case, I learned the refrigerator was a substitute for love. By seeking real honest affection, I got more satisfaction than I ever could from a piece of cheesecake.

Your Compulsion Replacement Chart

LIST YOUR COMPULSIONS AND THEN LIST REPLACEMENTS

AREA OF LIFE	COMPULSION	REPLACEMENT
Home (general)		
Work		
Social life		
Family		

Church life		
Free time		
Nighttime		
Meal time		

Do I want it just because it's there?
(My "ah hah" moment)

During my years as a chef and caterer, I had the opportunity to work in a gourmet deli. I was surrounded on all sides by every mouth-watering treat you could imagine and I gobbled them all up. Talk about a kid in a candy store! With hedonistic abandon, I indulged and tasted everything. It was my job to fill the enormous glass deli case with platters of fabulous entrees, salads, side dishes, and desserts. My boss, Marguerite Henderson (author of the cookbook *Savor the Memories*), was an unusually patient kitchen director because she put up with my wild cravings and frequent mistakes. She was also a kindred "foodie" with great enthusiasm for testing new recipes. Like a mad scientist, I dreamed up my every food fantasy and then experimented until each creation met with the sublime.

I merely had to ask and she would stock the walk-in cooler with beautiful radicchio for grilling or halibut for stuffing with tomatoes, olives, and prosciutto. If I wanted to glaze asparagus with garlic-balsamic vinegar and sprinkle it with roasted pine nuts—no problem. Skewered pork loin with a ginger-hoisan sauce and dried cherries? I gave it a whirl. My signature dish was roasted fillet of salmon with teriyaki caramel and sesame rice. Particularly mouth-watering were the lemon-blueberry scones with a buttermilk glaze (see *Recipes*).

Pretty much everywhere I looked there was fantastic food to sample. In fact, it was part of my job to taste, correct flavors, and taste again. Much of my true culinary education came from experiences I had in that kitchen. But even more valuable than on-the-job kitchen training was the life-changing realization that came two months into that experience. As I was preparing sheets of puff pastry stuffed with ham, gruyere cheese, Dijon mustard, and fresh thyme, my co-worker asked if I was hungry for a plate of gooey lasagna, hot from the oven. Normally hunger had nothing to do with whether or not I ate, but the truth was I just wasn't hungry and I acknowledged as much with refreshing honesty.

For the first time in my life, I chose to decline the lasagna—based on what I needed rather than what my mouth wanted. Then I took the next logical step: just because the chocolate truffle samples were sitting right there, I didn't need to eat them either. No matter how wonderful the barbecue chicken legs with corn pudding and garlic potato logs may have looked, I didn't have to eat them right at that moment. I could say: *"I don't want them because I don't need them."* No one was denying me anything I wanted, I was refusing it; and in that liberating act, I had an *"ah hah"* moment. Food lost its power over me that day. I realized I could choose my food instead of feeding the compulsion I had tended for 30 years. I came to the realization what I needed was what I wanted, instead of the other way around.

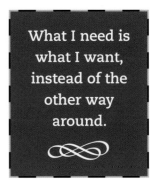

What I need is what I want, instead of the other way around.

When now presented with food, I ask, *"Am I hungry and do I really want to eat right now?"* instead of, *"There's a piece of mushroom pizza in the fridge so, I will put it in my mouth."* One empowers me to choose, the other enslaves me.

Be Wasteful

As you clean up the kitchen, do you eat the last of your kid's sandwich so it doesn't go to waste? At a restaurant, do you get your money's worth by finishing off your plate, even if you felt full during the salad course? If there is only one handful of chips left in the bag, is it too small to put back into the pantry—so you just eat it? Do you add the last three raviolis to your portion so you won't have to bother finding a container for the leftovers?

Let it go and throw it away. My Mom used to say, *"Better it go to waste than to your waist."* She was right. Shake off guilt for wasting food. If you think wasting food is irresponsible, listen up. You are more irresponsible when you compulsively shove excess food in your body than you are when you choose to scrape it into the sink. Consider your responsibility to your body and to your loved ones. It is nearly impossible to teach healthy habits without modeling them yourself. You are paramount—not those leftover peas. Food is just food. It doesn't have feelings. But you do. Food doesn't feel left out if you leave it on the plate. Be the master, not the slave.

Food is just food. It doesn't have feelings. But you do.

There Are No Bad Foods

Despite my general avoidance of hydrogenate fats and high-fructose corn syrup, there are no bad foods. Chocolate cake is our friend. Obviously, eating the entire cake in one sitting is not a wise move, but, when you need a treat, sharing a slice of chocolate decadence torte with a friend won't throw you off balance one bit. Preservatives, coloring agents, carbonated beverages, red meat, processed meats like hams or sausages, and pesticide-laden produce are not even bad foods, unless you ingest them with enough frequency to make them a significant part of your regular diet. Once a year, a Twinkie™ won't kill you. What you do most regularly defines you—hence, a diet of fresh veggies, whole grains, and excellent proteins, with an occasional toaster pastry, will define you as a healthy person.

I can eat all the food on the earth, just not in one day.

Say this one aloud as you try the *Rule of Halves* in Chapter 3: *"I can eat all the food on earth, just not in one day."* Truly, you can eat everything you want. Every yummy thing is available. Taking away restrictions is a mighty freedom. It allows us to see food in an impartial way because we are not hanging onto it with a deathlike grip anymore. We have our whole

> **TIP 17**
>
> **Eat a Brownie with Broccoli.** *When you do enjoy a treat, eat it that day in combination with other high value foods. This gives you the nutrition to use up those carbohydrates and fat for fuel.*

lives to enjoy the delicious bounty of the world—even those *occasional* foods we simply cannot live without. If your body tells you it does not need a treat, it could mean your meals are already rich with fats, sugar, and salt. So, if you want the nod from your bod to eat a fine chocolate truffle in the afternoon, choose a lighter lunch—think salad.

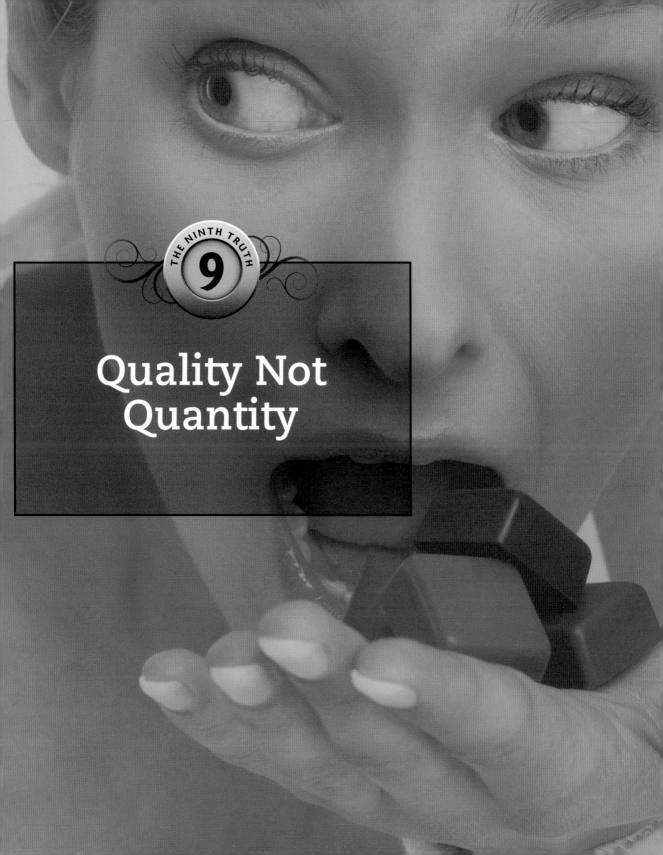

THE NINTH TRUTH

9

Quality Not
Quantity

It takes good fuel to encourage a metabolism to burn fat.
This chapter provides a closer look at what we should eat
regularly and what foods are best enjoyed occasionally.

Minimize Unsubstantial Carbohydrates

Carbohydrates are nutrients that give us energy. There are primarily two kinds of carbohydrates: simple and complex. Simple carbohydrates give you energy quickly. They can be absorbed almost immediately because they rapidly turn to sugar in the bloodstream. White sugar, cake, and white bread are good examples of foods built with simple carbs. They also raise your insulin production (which regulates blood sugar) very quickly. The problem with excessive simple carbs is you probably won't be able to expend all the sugar energy you've ingested. And what do you do with that leftover energy? It is either stored as glycogen in your cells (which are probably at full glycogen capacity already) or stored as fat. Minimize these unsubstantial carbohydrates by replacing them with complex carbohydrates—whole grains and fewer sugars (*Christian & Greger, 110-136*).

Complex carbohydrates take longer to increase blood sugar levels, but they maintain your energy longer and taper off slowly. Some examples of complex carbs include: whole grain bread, oatmeal, flaxseed, nuts, yams, beans, peas, barley, quinoa, and brown rice. These foods also feature fiber, which gives you clearer skin, fewer illnesses, reduced body odor, better breath, shinier hair, and better vascular health to increase optimal sexual performance. Clearly, fiber is not just for the elderly. Not only does fiber help maintain normal bowel movements while it scrubs your intestinal track clean as a whistle, but it has a tempering effect on insulin demand.

To compare the effects of simple verses complex carbohydrates, let's pretend you drink a can of soda—which contains as much as sixteen teaspoons of sugar; a lot of simple carbohydrates. Soda spikes the body's insulin production while it quickly raises blood sugar levels. You feel a sugar boost after drinking it, but that soon peaks and drops away just as fast, leaving you "droopy." On the other hand, a bowl of whole grain oatmeal contains complex carbohydrates (and lots of fiber which slows absorption), thereby providing steadier energy that lasts longer. Complex carbohydrates also require a steady delivery of less insulin, helping prevent overuse of our overworked pancreas—ground zero for diabetes. Normal bowel movements, clean intestines, and reduced risk of diabetes—all for the low price of oats. Can you beat that!

SIMPLE CARBOHYDRATES

☹ Excess sugars to store as fat
☹ Little nutritive value
☹ Insulin spike

COMPLEX CARBOHYDRATES

☺ Usable energy
☺ Essential nutrition (including fiber)
☺ Moderate insulin demand

Fruit is a potent source of vitamins, fiber, and antioxidants. Although fruit contains natural sugars, they are less concentrated than say, candy. So, fruit should be eaten daily, in small amounts.

And let's not forget our vegetables. Most vegetables contain large amounts of fiber, minimal sugar, and are packed with nutrients, so we need to build our meals around them. Include lean protein when your body prompts you to do so. Meat should be consumed only as

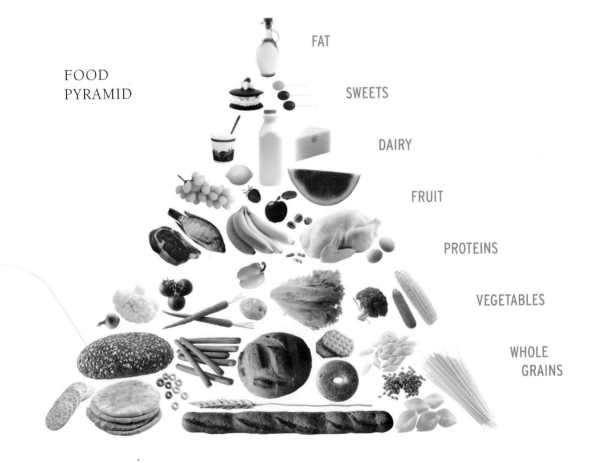

FOOD
PYRAMID

FAT

SWEETS

DAIRY

FRUIT

PROTEINS

VEGETABLES

WHOLE
GRAINS

needed—more in cold weather, less in warm weather (see the section below on *Climate and Meat*). We also require more protein after greater amounts of physical activity than during times of inactivity. Beef, pork, lamb, and cheese contain varying degrees of saturated fat, so don't base your diet on hamburgers, ribs, and cheese sandwiches. Proteins like beans, fish, chicken, tofu, eggs, and nuts are healthy and should take a more prominent role in your diet. Dairy is loaded with nutritional value like vitamin D and calcium. But, dairy products also contain animal fat and sugar—which means careful portion control is a must. Bottom line: anchor your diet in whole grains and vegetables, with fruit, meat, and dairy added as needed. It seems like Mom was right all along.

Sugar & White Flour

Consider reducing sugar from your daily routine—not completely, but as a general rule. A surprising amount of added sugars are hidden in foods we think of as "healthy" such as: peanut butter, yogurt, breakfast cereals, breakfast bars, granola bars, canned fruit, applesauce, gelatin, fruit snacks, fruit juices, and energy drinks. Other sugar-intensive foods include: jam, ketchup, barbecue sauce, baked goods, soup mixes, puddings, frozen treats, milk chocolate, and almost every pre-packaged, processed food on the planet.

If you love something sweet, go for homemade treats like cookies or brownies because they generally contain less sugar than store-bought varieties. One of my favorite low-sugar snacks is strawberries (or bananas) dipped in sour cream and then dipped in crushed semi-sweet chocolate chips, nuts, and a sprinkling of brown sugar. Our tastes adapt as we adjust to less-intensely sweet desserts. Over time, orange slices drizzled with honey and sprinkled with cinnamon will be preferable over a candy bar.

Try to replace white flour with whole grain flour. The term *whole wheat* means the flour includes the bran or outer membrane of the grain. White flour is pervasive in our Western diet, but, with a little effort, you can select sandwiches with whole grain bread and discover other whole grain options. Be careful to not be fooled by clever labels. 100% wheat flour is still refined *white* flour. The label must read *100% whole wheat* flour in order to qualify as a whole grain food. In most wheat bread you will find a combination of white and whole grain flour. Remember, the more whole grain, the better.

Common white flour foods to watch out for include: rolls, buns, tortillas, crackers, pancakes, pastry, breakfast bars, pasta, baked treats (muffins, cookies, sweet rolls, pastries, etc.), pizza crust, salty snacks (like pretzels and chips), and some breakfast cereals. White flour is also used as a thickener in a wide variety of processed foods like soups, sauces, and prepared frozen and packaged meals.

Does this mean you will never get to eat a stack of pancakes again? Of course not, because your normal diet dictates your health, not the exceptions. If you regularly eat a whole grain breakfast (see *Tammy's Granola* in the recipe section), or other breakfast like: eggs, unsweetened yogurt with a bit of fruit mixed in, wheat toast, fruit, etc., and then once a year you enjoy the 4th of July fire department pancake breakfast, you will stay balanced. As an aside, if your body asks for pancakes more than once a year, fulfill your cravings at home with good quality whole grain pancakes—make your own or buy a good mix. Should you go out and purchase a grain mill to grind your own wheat? Sure, if you want to, and if you do, you have my admiration because anything made from freshly ground flour is an ethereal experience. But if you are not so inclined (like me), start reading labels to find whole grain bread and pancake mix.

Minimize Excess Animal Fat

Fat must first be stored before it can be used as energy. Unlike carbohydrates, it doesn't break down into sugar and go whizzing through our bodies as energy. No, fat is sugar's slow, stupid cousin. It seeps its viscous self into our cells, which happily balloon and expand as they get crowded. If we don't require our cells to surrender fat as fuel (by exercising), fat stays quite comfortable on our hips for years.

There are basically two types of fat, saturated and unsaturated. You have probably heard about healthful oils. These fall into the unsaturated category and come from plants, nuts, and seeds like corn, canola, and olive oil. They reduce bad cholesterol (the artery clogging kind) and some contain elements essential to the body like those found in sunflower oil, safflower oil, nuts, and oily fish. However, all oils are high in calories and need to be portion controlled. We do require a certain amount of fat to be healthy, but there is enough fat in a piece of chicken to meet that requirement for several days. If you are an omnivore and you eat dairy products there is little risk you will expire of insufficient fat consumption.

Saturated fats are the ones we want to replace. They mostly come from animals and dairy products. They are non-essential to the body and they increase the production of cholesterol in our arteries—posing a health risk to our hearts. Saturated fats also block the benefits of healthful unsaturated oils.

You know your oil is saturated when it solidifies at room temperature. Think about the thick, white stuff left in the bottom of the pan after cooking bacon; this is the fat you want to avoid. Animal fat is found in processed meats (sausages, hot dogs, deli meats), butter (ah yes, my beloved butter), lard, and in cake mixes, piecrust, and biscuits. Although derived from plants, palm oil and coconut oil are also saturated and should be limited. There are many good oils available on the market and it is easy to find healthful substitutes. For cooking, I enjoy canola and olive oil. For flavorful salads dressings, try walnut, flaxseed, extra-virgin olive, and rapeseed oil.

Hydrogenated Fats and Trans Fatty Acids (Trans Fats)

As mentioned earlier, one of the foods I would caution against altogether, it is shortening. Shortening is made from hydrogenated fat. Hydrogenated fats are oils chemically altered so their molecules no longer take a liquid form. Hydrogenation straightens the molecules so they pack closer together, resulting in thick fat that is firm at room temperature. This is what makes shortening solid instead of runny (*Wolke, 71-72*).

This process of hydrogenation, the forcing of hydrogen into the fat molecule, also creates the dreaded trans fatty acids, also called trans fats. They raise your "bad LDL" cholesterol and lower your "good HDL" cholesterol levels. In a nutshell, the process of partial hydrogenation or full hydrogenation changes the position of the hydrogen atom, making the unsaturated oil molecule resemble that of a saturated fat molecule (think bacon grease). Your body then treats the changed fat as if it were bacon grease. The health implications of trans fats are pretty serious, with heart disease, stroke, diabetes, and obesity as the major threats. Since 2006, the FDA has required manufacturers to separately list trans fatty acids on labels, but even without looking for it you can be sure trans fats are in just about every commercially fried food and convenience store snack (*Wolke, 166-171*).

Naturally, manufacturers of your favorite snack cake are trying ride the tide of public opinion by staying under the FDA's limit of 0.5 gram per serving so their packaging can read: "*Contains No Trans Fatty Acids.*" However, it still contains some trans fat, even if it is only a small amount. Another tricky label to watch for is: "*Made with 100% pure vegetable oils.*" What that advertising does not say is whether or not their cooking oil has been hydrogenated. Your restaurant kitchen probably gets its cooking fat in a semi-solid form, all the while advertising the use of 100% unsaturated oils. How do they get around these semantics? Hydrogenated fat can be made from vegetable oil and can, therefore, be touted as such, whereas, it is unnecessary to hydrogenate most saturated fats because they are already firm at room temperature—typically known as lard.

Our bodies cope as well as they can with altered fat molecules such as shortening. They store the fat, manufacture cholesterol in our arteries, block the benefits of the almonds and salmon we eat, and thoroughly get gummed up. And hydrogenated fat is EVERYWHERE. In addition to headlining as plain old shortening, it is found in (get ready): margarine, soup mixes, most fast food, some restaurant food, frozen hash browns, breakfast cereal, tortillas, potato chips, crackers, ramen noodles, frozen whipped topping, ice cream, gravy mixes, biscuit mix, peanut butter, cake mix, roasted nuts, cheese spreads, pastries, doughnuts, muffins, chocolate milk, coffee creamer, chocolate candy coatings, frosting, and almost every processed kids food on the market, just to name a few! If it comes from a pop-out tube or from a box, it probably has hydrogenated fat in it. The best chance of eliminating hydrogenated fat from your diet is to make food yourself from scratch or seek out alternatives without hydrogenated fat. For instance, instead of chips and dip, have whole-wheat pita triangles with purchased hummus. Instead of peanut butter with hydrogenated fat, look for the "natural" varieties of peanut butter made from only peanuts and salt. If you must have a brownie, make it yourself with healthy oil instead of using a mix.

Avoid cooking with margarine; it is typically made from hydrogenated fat and it usually contains an unknown quantity of water which affects its cooking properties. Try to cook in olive oil with just a touch of butter for flavor. I prefer butter over margarine because its natural form is more recognizable to my system. Sure, butter is a saturated fat and should be portion controlled, but at least it is not hydrogenated fat full of trans fatty acids. Make it easy on your body to use fat for fuel. Eat healthful oils and avoid hydrogenated fats.

Fried Food

Eat fried foods sparingly. They are usually cooked in hydrogenated fats, and sometimes saturated hydrogenated fats. After a bacon burger (yes, the bacon is usually deep fried) and a side order of cheese fries, you might as well get out the heart-attack paddles. But to put things in perspective, I might eat fried calamari or tempura vegetables twice a year because, let's face it, a girl's gotta live. Otherwise, I don't indulge in deep fried food. Hydrogenated fat is still the primary frying fat in commercial use. Your favorite restaurant's fried chicken is probably loaded with shortening. Furthermore, even if it is cooked in healthy oil rather than hydrogenated fat, high heat has a damaging effect on oil. Even polyunsaturated and monounsaturated oils, like sunflower or corn, lose their healthful benefits when they reach the 400-450 degrees required for deep-frying. There are some indicators that, at 430-degrees, oil molecules can change on a chemical level and become carcinogenic. So, limit your intake of fried food, replacing it with lean meats, seafood, and vegetables sautéed in healthful oil. Sautéed food requires less oil and gentler heat because direct contact with the pan cooks the food instead of the blistering heat of deep fry oil. I recommend olive or canola oil for sautéing because they have such a high flash point they resist decomposition (no smoking oil).

So, what should you eat?

Real Food

We have talked a bit about which foods to avoid. Let's talk about what you want to enjoy more of. All food is good, but start eating *real food*, or non-processed food, meaning food products as close to their original form as possible. For instance, a scrambled egg with salsa, a ripe peach and a slice of whole-wheat toast with butter is more recognizable to your system than a purchased breakfast burrito. It probably takes about the same amount of time to prepare the first option as it does to go through the drive-through or microwave the frozen alternative. Limit processed or commercially prepared food as much as possible, choosing instead healthy *real food* options.

Whole grains

Load your body with the quality fuel of whole grains. We know soluble oat bran fiber lowers blood cholesterol and lowers glucose metabolism in diabetes patients because it prevents insulin spikes. Researchers also believe bran may help prevent certain types of cancer. But don't go overboard and start dumping ten spoonfuls of bran on your cereal in the morning. Excess fiber can result in gassy intestinal irritation and its health benefits may only be realized from eating bran-rich food rather than from piling little bran shavings on your plate. Daily servings of whole grain breads and cereals will do the job just fine.

With a little imagination, it is easy to incorporate new varieties into your diet. Try using whole grains in place of rice, noodles, or potatoes.

Taste the sweet

Learn to taste naturally occurring sweetness. Even bitter foods carry underlying tones of sweet which is a benefit because bitter foods and unsweetened drinks help arrest cravings without adding unneeded calories, sugars, or unhealthy fats to your balanced day. Do not sweeten foods with synthetic sweeteners—it simply perpetuates an unnatural need for excessive sweetening in your food. If you are not yet a fan of bitter flavors, try a fine quality dark chocolate and really taste it. You might be surprised at the sweet notes that balance out the sharp bitter in chocolate. In fact, there are sweet notes in most of our food if we are willing to tune in and taste. For instance, unsweetened milk is quite sweet. Lemons contain as much sugar as an orange, but their high citric acid concentration blitzes our taste buds before we detect the sugar. Try and see if you can taste the sweet in lemons. Carrots, red bell peppers, tomatoes (on the vine), onions, and yams are incredibly sweet. Even white rice has notes of sweet on the tongue. Raw food simply prepared, without commercial processing, reveals true flavors—including sweetness you may be unaware of.

Lean Proteins

Fish, seafood, eggs, turkey, chicken, tofu, yogurt, low-fat varieties of cheese, nuts and nut-butters, seeds, and beans are all delicious forms of lean protein. Try to adjust your diet to include, primarily, these proteins with occasional departures into red meat territory. Beef stroganoff or a pepperoni pizza twice a year will not kill you, but your day-to-day input

Try New Grains. Quinoa (keen-wah) is an ancient grain thought to have been a staple of the Mayan diet. It is one of the most protein-rich and fiber-rich grains on the planet. Its tiny, coiled particles taste pleasantly nutty and cook up just like rice. Try preparing it in a rice cooker with a dab of butter. Throw whole grains like quinoa into soups and stews for added texture and nutrition. Use cooked and cooled grains in cold middle-eastern salads, like tabouli. To make tabouli, simply toss the cooked grains with chopped parsley, tomatoes, garlic, lemon juice, and olive oil. Serve over greens or alongside grilled chicken. See the Tabouli recipe at the end of the book for more detailed instructions.

Kamut, buckwheat, and spelt are cousins to wheat with terrific taste and texture possibilities. Try baking your own bread with these grains. Baking connects us to the basics in life, cathartically working out stresses while sustaining us. Even if you don't bake often, reward yourself with the opportunity as often as you need it, and don't be afraid to try new kinds of flour milled from whole grains. Add sprouted grains to pancakes, baked goods, and yogurt (see below for sprouting instructions). When soaked overnight, most whole grains can also be cooked into a delicious, and inexpensive, morning breakfast cereal.

Barley is an ancient grain that fueled the mighty Spartan warriors of old. They were called "barley eaters" because their size and stamina was built on a diet of barley gruel. When cooked "al dente," barley is firm with a bite and makes for an excellent pilaf alongside any meat entrée—simply cook it in flavored cooking liquid (like vegetable stock) and stir in seasonings like saffron and garlic. Barley is the foundation for great risotto when simmered with shallots, herbs, chicken stock, and white wine. In soups, barley takes on a tender texture while absorbing the flavors of the broth. Use it as you would rice or pasta. See more barley recipes in the recipe section at the end of this book.

Amaranth, corn, oats, whole-wheat couscous, and many other grains provide delicious alternatives to the basic American diet of noodles, potatoes, or white rice. "Try them, try them, and you may..." (Dr. Suess, 53)

Sprouted Grains. To sprout grains, soak them at room temperature for six hours. Drain, and allow grains to sit unattended overnight on the counter. In the morning, observe the tiny little shoots emerging from each kernel. Sprouted grains are incredibly healthy and make a nice addition to bread dough and cereal.

should come from healthier options. You may find it easy to do. Ground turkey can substitute for hamburger in almost any recipe. A peanut butter sandwich (made from 100% ground peanuts with no added hydrogenated fat) on whole wheat bread wins the prize as the easiest and least expensive lunch option. Try a quintessential French salad of fried egg over mixed greens with a drizzle of lemon juice and olive oil—bright flavors, healthy and inexpensive! How does roasted salmon with pesto sauce and sautéed green beans with sweet peppers sound? Yum! Or, perhaps you might be surprised to enjoy a fantastic *Tofu Stir-fry with Broccoli and Mushrooms* (see Recipes). Choose leaner protein options based on your needs and also on the weather. The following section discusses a rarely-examined aspect of health management—adjusting our diet with the climate.

Climate & Meat

When the weather is warm, we require less meat. Why is this? During balmy weather our bodies don't need to work as hard to maintain a constant body temperature. On the flip side, throughout history, animal fats have been crucial to surviving cold months, when winter restricted our ability to grow and forage food. Meat contains essential vitamins that would be otherwise absent from the diet when fruit and vegetable stores were gone. Added layers of body fat also meant warmth.

Because we now have central heating and access to grocery store vegetables throughout winter, we may not need nearly as much meat as our ancestors required. Additionally, our basic biological need for meat is diminished in warm climates and hot weather, despite the fact that hot dogs and steaks on the "barbie" are a long-standing tradition at the summer picnic. If garbanzo beans on a salad with avocado, lemon juice, and olive oil will keep you in balance, don't also add meat out of habit. Consume meat every few days or so, based on your activity and metabolism. When it gets colder, your body may tell you to transition back to daily servings of meat protein. Pay attention to your body and climate changes. For a tasty alternative to meat try the *Garden Burger* recipe in the recipe section at the end of this book.

Lots of Colors on Your Plate

Consider your plate as if it were a light spectrum wheel. Ideally, it should have many colors on it—like a light wheel. A lone frozen burrito may be "dinner" to some, but it won't fuel a high-performance metabolism. You need more color because colors indicate "high-octane" fuel. Add to that burrito some sliced tomatoes, baby spinach, shredded green and purple cabbage, an avocado slice, a carrot stick, fresh salsa with onions, peppers, and cilantro, a dollop of whole milk yogurt or sour cream, and a wedge of a juicy orange, and let's see, how many other colors could we possibly pack on the plate?

The more colors, the more likely you will consume a balanced amount of different foods with all the nutritional power you need.

Raw Food

When food is cooked, it loses alkalinity and its PH balance becomes more acidic. Eating raw plant food (like lettuce) raises the alkalinity PH of our cells. Some studies indicate that when human cells are more alkaline, they are better able to fight disease and aging (*Brotman & Lenkert*). The typical American diet has an extremely high acidic PH, as a direct result of cooked meats, fats, caffeine, sugar, and alcohol. Interestingly, our obesity epidemic is linked to these same elements.

There is a whole raw food movement in this country, complete with raw food restaurants and "uncook" books—see *The Raw Gourmet by Nomi Shannon*. Because moderation is the key to lifelong health, a completely raw diet is too extreme to be part of my balanced lifestyle. Don't get me wrong, I believe in the benefits of raw food. I enjoy something raw every day. But, going on a 100% raw kick is a perfect example of an unsustainable diet. While most of us cannot and will not adhere to a completely raw diet, the prudence of including raw food in every meal just seems smart. It is easy to add a fresh piece of fruit or vegetable to each meal. Salads loaded with beautiful crunchy things and succulent fruity things are a normal part of any balanced, and alkaline, diet. Even school lunchrooms and fast food drive-thrus usually offer carrot and celery sticks or apple slices. In short, add a piece of fresh fruit to your breakfast, load down your sandwich with veggies at lunch, and enjoy some raw items as part of your "color wheel" at dinner.

Hydration

Our bodies are made primarily of water. Yet, most of us remain in a chronic state of dehydration. Proper hydration is an obvious requirement to stay balanced. Fluids carry away toxins, flush our bowels, improve circulation, and feed oxygen to our brains, just to name a few benfits. Good stuff…water. I prefer water at a cool room temperature without ice. If ice in your water bottle is the only way you can suck it down, then keep the ice. However, according to traditional Asian medicine, the intense cold of ice interrupts the healthy flow of energy (chi), preventing some of the health benefits of water. Regardless of the temperature, drink more water.

In fact, the next time you feel a bit peckish for salty or sweet snacks, try a tall glass of water. Chances are those cravings mean thirst, rather than hunger. Get in the habit of drinking water before raiding the crackers. See Tip #2 on page 23. One of the first symptoms of minor dehydration is a headache. Treat headaches first with a tall glass of water. During a menstrual cycle, hydration is the first line of defense against cramps and bloating. Feeling tired? Take a big drink. Keeping water on hand makes it easier to hydrate throughout the day. The following tips should help you increase your water intake:

TIP 18

Don't Drink Your Calories. Many Americans consume up to 40% of their daily calories by drinking sugary beverages. This includes soda, coffee drinks, sweetened tea, juices, energy drinks, and sports drinks. Even 100% fruit juice, although it contains vitamins, can contain large concentrations of natural sugar. Limit juice portion to 6-ounces or less per day. Cut the extra calories you won't particularly miss and save your calories for the food you want. Drink water. You need it.

Ways to Hydrate

- Keep a water bottle in the car with you, or in your handbag.

- Substitute water for soda, coffee drinks, fruit juices, energy drinks, or sports drinks.

- During exercise, take frequent water breaks.

- Get a hot/cold water cooler in your house.

- Install a water purification filter on your faucet.

- Every time you get a headache, feel fatigue, have cramps, or experience a craving, take a big drink of water.

- Combat nighttime grazing with a warm cup of herb tea or a non-caffeinated coffee substitute like *Pero®* barley and malt beverage. Add lemon or milk for a sleep-inducing finish to your day. When taken slightly bitter, warm drinks can stop further cravings and close the palette.

- Splurge on yummy herb teas.

- Use pretty glassware and garnish water with a slice of lemon, cucumber, or strawberry.

Foods in Season

Tune in to your body and you will discover natural cycles and seasons. We experience daily, monthly, and yearly physical changes. Yes, even men have cycles. Everything in nature is designed around seasonal changes therefore it makes sense that our bodies have seasonal requirements as well. To apply this to our food choices, seek out food in season. The earth provides what we need when we need it. The vitamin C in oranges and strawberries happens to come during winter and spring, exactly when our tired immune systems need it the most. When in-season, plants produce their sweetest crop. Sure, you can find greenhouse-grown items yearlong, but peak-season fruit and vegetables are more flavorful and nutritious.

Not only does produce taste better in season, it is far less expensive. During my first pregnancy, I paid over $15.00 for honeydew melon in February. It tasted blah, and wasn't even sweet. In August, far superior-tasting melons cost as little as $2.00 each. It makes sense to enjoy peas in spring, corn in July, peaches in August, and greens throughout the year.

From an economic standpoint, it is beneficial to yourself and others to support the growers of your area by buying local. Purchase from farmers markets and fruit stands when available. Look on the stickers at the grocery store for the origin of that watermelon. The less time it spends on a truck, the more time it can spend on the vine developing sweetness. Buying seasonally and locally not only guarantees better taste and prices, it also helps support small-scale farming of heirloom varieties. Commercial farms grow only those varieties that hold up well to transportation. Lots of old-time varieties have been phased out in favor of new hybrids that produce a higher yield with longer shelf life. Supporting smaller farms means older (better tasting) varieties will continue to be in demand. It might just be your neighbor selling herbs at the farmers market so get up early and go support them while you feed your engine the fuel it needs today.

If you need help remembering the growing season for various plants, I recommend websites like *foodnetwork.com* and *epicurious.com* for ongoing seasonal food discussions and recipes. The following chart on page 122, printed with permission from www.gardenshare. org, is an excellent seasonal food guide (Copyright (C) 2005 GardenShare Inc.). It features seasonal plant availabilities in the northern half of the United States. Warmer southern states have multiple growing seasons for some plants; so, Southerners can also use the chart, with the knowledge that radishes and beans will come around again in only a few months.

Learn To Cook a Little and Eat Well

Become proficient at cooking the foods that make you feel well. At a minimum, select seven healthy dishes you like and practice them until you can make one for each night of the week. Your repertoire should match the medical needs of those you cook for, and meet the time

EATING WITH THE SEASONS
IN THE
NORTH COUNTRY

Suggestions to Help You Eat Local Food Throughout the Year

JANUARY

Grass-fed beef
Goat cheese

From storage:
Winter squash
Onions, garlic
Potatoes, turnips, rutabagas

From the freezer:
Apple cider
Homemade pesto
Garden vegetables

FEBRUARY

Chicken
Bison
Hazelberts

From the pantry:
Honey
Home-canned tomatoes, applesauce,
sauerkraut, pickles, fruit, jams & jellies

Grow your own sprouts

MARCH

Maple syrup
Dry beans

From the pantry:
Dried herbal teas, vinegars
Dried tomatoes

From the garden:
Dig parsnips, salsify

Make your own yogurt

APRIL

Eggs
Cheese

From field & stream:
Wild leeks

From the coldframe & greenhouse:
Spinach, arugula, greens

From the garden:
Dig horseradish

MAY

Spinach
Sorrel
Asparagus
Rhubarb

From field & garden:
Fiddleheads
Wild orpine
Dandelion greens
Chives, green onions

JUNE

Lettuce & greens
Asparagus
Rhubarb
Peas
Strawberries
Tomatoes (maybe!)

From the wild:
Elderberries, blackcaps

Visit the farmer's markets

JULY

Tomatoes
Peas
Strawberries, blueberries, raspberries
Gooseberries, currants, Juneberries
Cherries
Garlic
Carrots
New potatoes
Fresh herbs

U-pick, U-eat

AUGUST

Sweet corn
Tomatoes, peppers, eggplant
Early apples
Blueberries
Melons
Onions
Carrots
Basil, cilantro

Farm stands & gardens overflowing!

SEPTEMBER

Apples
Raspberries
Melons
Onions
Potatoes

From the roadside:
Wild grape jelly

Last chance:
Tomatoes, peppers, eggplant

OCTOBER

Venison
Apples, fresh cider
Pumpkins
Raspberries
Brussels sprouts
Cabbage for making sauerkraut

From the garden:
Leeks, celeriac, kohlrabi
Collard & beet greens
Salads: mâche, claytonia

NOVEMBER

Turkey
Venison
Apples

From storage:
Cabbage
Winter squash

From the garden:
Kale
Jerusalem artichokes

DECEMBER

From storage:
Potatoes, turnips, rutabagas
Onions, garlic
Dried tomatoes

From the garden:
Kale
Carrots (mulched)

Bake your own bread

Copyright © 2005 GardenShare Inc.
www.GardenShare.org

constraints of your life. For instance, if members of your family are on a low-sodium, low-cholesterol diet, practice dishes that meet those needs. Consult websites and cookbooks to meet that requirement. If you have only thirty minutes each day to make good food, choose dishes you like that are quick and easy to prepare. Crock-pots are a boon to families because in the morning food goes in the pot, and when your troops are hungry hot food comes out. Feel free to find new ideas from the recipes at the end of this book. They are notated to indicate which recipes are quick (thirty minutes or under), healthy ("daily fuel" as opposed to "occasional treats"), kid friendly, vegetarian, and inexpensive.

Experiment until you find several flavor profiles you enjoy. For instance, I like anything cooked with garlic, ginger, and soy sauce. I also like the combination of mushrooms, onions, Dijon mustard, and thyme. Plug-in your favorite flavor profiles with food your body is craving. You *do not* have to be a chef to feed yourself well. You just need to place enough value on your health to make the effort.

To improve your cooking skills read books and magazines. Take a basic community education cooking class. Good food does not require expensive equipment. You can produce most meals with a soup pot, a fry pan, and a flexible cutting board. Buy a salad spinner and a non-serrated chef's knife. If you haven't used your kitchen in a while, call your Mom and ask her which is a pot and which is a pan. Can you use a chef's knife or a carrot peeler properly? If not, prepping fresh fruits and vegetables is not only tiresome, it can be dangerous to your fingers (for knife-handling tips, read the following section). If learning to feed yourself sounds onerous, take heart. Reading one issue of *Bon Appetit*™ magazine from cover to cover every few months will help you become adequately equipped with both method and inspiration. You don't like gourmet food? Try the yummy recipes in the *Fannie Farmer Cookbook*© and the *Fannie Farmer Baking Book*©. For those who want an upper level immersion course, read the *Joy of Cooking, by Rombauer and Becker*©. If you don't like to cook, think of it this way: if your boss asked you to manage a vital area of your organization, and all you had to do was read a magazine once every couple of months, would you balk? You are the organization and your body is vital. Keep it simple because we have other demands in our lives. Perhaps take fifteen minutes per day to discover ways to improve your family's diet. It will take time but it will pay off. Read and then cook!

To increase your cooking abilities try out farmers markets and specialty stores in your area. Talk to the produce person in your grocery store. Become familiar with unfamiliar foods by trying them. Do not be afraid of rutabagas or jicama or broccoli sprouts or oat groats. If a vegetable looks good but you don't have the slightest idea how to prepare it, ask Mr. Produce guy at your market. Or search the internet for recipes and suggestions (see www.epicurious.com).

Ease in gently with changes in diet. If your family is used to eating Hot Pockets™ they might not immediately cheer at the presentation of a broccoli-cheese frittata.

In the event you have been living in a fallout shelter for the last twenty years and you don't know the basic nutritional values of food—such as grapefruits have vitamin C, and milk has calcium—get a book and read. Try filling a spare minute perusing *Prevention©* magazine. Every issue contains relevant information packaged in a user-friendly way. It might sound droll, but learning about the weight loss benefits of figs and the heart benefits of almonds perks up my interest every time. If you take seriously the charge to manage your body, to treat it like a Ferrari®, you will want all the information available to fulfill that stewardship.

Knife-Handling

Become adept with a chef's knife to speed up the prep of fruit and vegetables. Step-by-step instructions on how to use your knife like a pro can be found at www.cheftalk.com or on www.youtube.com. Search the key words: *How to use a chef's knife* to find endless help on the internet. Once you master knife technique, it is easy to quickly prep fresh ingredients. As a note: knives are sharp. Please adhere to safe knife-handling practices and use common sense when cooking to avoid accidents.

Cook for Yourself

Cooking takes time. Perhaps it isn't feasible every day. It requires access to a kitchen and, heaven forbid, grocery shopping. Of course individual situations vary, but try to prepare your own food as much as you can. We can better fuel our bodies when we control what ends up on our plates. Eating out at restaurants is convenient and tastes good, but the reason restaurant food tastes indulgent is because it contains more fat, salt, white flour, and sugar than food we cook at home—not to mention it is expensive!

As you cook for the family, cook for yourself. Do not fix different meals for different tastes. That is just plain crazy. You could spend all your time and money accommodating each picky eater in the family. Think of *one meal for everybody* as tough love at the table. With time, the entire family will become accustomed to your tastes and preferences. How do I know? Millions of kids in Asia eat dried seaweed for a snack. Kids in Italy eat zucchini blossoms stuffed with ricotta cheese. Kids in Spain put down fried squid without a thought. And my own children have decided mustard is not the yellow poison they once thought. My point: children learn to like the foods they are presented with. Eventually.

But how do I reconcile the policy of cooking for myself while encouraging my family to listen to their bodies and select the food they need? Won't my needs be different from my teenage daughter's? The answer is: portion size. If you provide lots of colors and essential foods in a meal, different family members can learn to take more or less of each item depending on their individual needs. For example, if they need more whole-wheat toast than you, they might take two pieces while you might choose only a half of a slice. If you need greens, you might load your plate with fresh spinach salad while others may balance out a small salad with a variety of other foods. Over time, as you mix up the frequency with which you choose fish, yogurt, yams, or green beans (or any food) you will generally match the needs of those you cook for because they will have access to foods they need and they will acclimate to your schedule.

One-Bite Rule

I once read a report that stated it takes over eighteen exposures to a new taste and texture for a child to accept a new food. Translate this into the *One-Bite Rule*, requiring every kid at the table (and reluctant grown-ups) to choke down at least one bite of each dish. After repeated exposures to sautéed mushrooms with garlic, their tastes mature and they might decide—"hey, that's pretty good."

Teaching Kids To Choose Well. Parents have the added responsibility to teach children to listen to their bodies. The following tips illustrate how it can be done with a little patience.

First, help them understand what a healthy meal contains. Show them what good food looks like, so they understand it does not necessarily come from a frozen package or with a cheap toy. Identify for them the ideal portion of protein, vegetable, grain or starch, fruit, dairy, and water. Demonstrate how to enjoy an appropriate treat. Share with them when your body prompts you to eat treats. And share with them when your body tells you to stop. Teach by example and discussion.

Second, ask them to really taste treats and share their discoveries. Is it too cold, too sweet, really creamy, full of buttery flavor, or just right?

Third, when kids want only pizza and ice cream, ask them what is missing from that menu. Ask them to enjoy green beans before having another handful of chips. Use questions to provoke their considerations of what does and does not constitute a balanced choice. Remember, if they don't learn this at home, they probably will not learn it. Ultimately, I recommend kids take lunch from home because it is almost impossible to avoid hydrogenated fats, high fructose corn syrup, and processed food in cafeterias.

Good, Better, and Best

I know most people cannot stop work to go home and whip up a three-course lunch, but take care of your needs the best you can. If you bring a lunch to work or school, prepare something worth eating. At home, invest in yourself and make each meal good for your engine—even if you have to peel a carrot and wash some lettuce. A toaster pastry will not fuel your Ferrari™ like a piece of leftover chicken on a bed of baby greens, avocado, and tomato. Throw in a handful of almonds and some yummy dressing and you have a lunch you can look forward to. If you live alone, give yourself permission to cook for one person. You don't have to prep a dinner party for eight in order to make something awesome. Scrambled eggs and broccoli with toast takes under 5 minutes to whip up, providing stellar nutrition.

When there is no time to grab something from home, order food as close to what you would have made if you had the opportunity. An apple can be found in most cafeterias. Half-portion sandwiches on whole grain bread, brothy vegetable soups, salads, grilled chicken, and fish options, without excessive sauces, will usually provide premium fuel for your tank. Vending machines generally do not sell anything your body asks for. But life happens and sometimes there is no other option—you have to bite the bullet and eat cheese puffs for lunch. Just try to fulfill your body's requests for high-grade fuel as regularly as possible. For most people, there is a *good, better, and best* option for meals. Make good-tasting *real food* important enough to choose the *best* option.

Map Your Store

Spend your time and money in the outer aisles of the store. These aisles are generally stocked with fresh fruits, veggies, dairy, meat, and bread. Avoid interior aisles displaying snacks, frozen food, boxed meals, canned prepared food, and processed mixes. Get in the habit of walking right by the soda and chips aisle. If you need a bag of frozen peas, don't linger in front of the whipped topping and ice cream. When you venture down the canned goods aisle for some chicken stock, marinara sauce, or garbanzo beans, don't loiter by the myriad of instant meals in a can. Try to purchase food in its non-processed form. For instance, instead of buying a can of chili with meat and beans (which can contain huge amounts of saturated animal fat and salt), simmer canned beans with ground turkey, tomatoes, chopped onions, chilies, and a spoonful of chili powder. It might take you an extra ten minutes to throw in the pan, but it is worth it. Use the suggested *Pantry Stock Guide* at the end of this book to keep items on hand that will help you cook the foods you love.

Eat the Highest Quality Food You Can Afford

Eat the highest quality food you can afford because it is fresher, seasonal, and less processed. It also means better texture and flavor. I am not suggesting we eat filet mignon and lobster tail at every meal—even if we could afford it. Nor am I advocating buying strictly organic. Although organic is better, it is sometimes not affordable or available, and frankly, sometimes it does not look as fresh. I am referring to buying local sweet corn on the cob or crunchy fall apples that may cost more than those shipped in from another continent—but are worth every penny. More flavor means increased satisfaction. More satisfaction means we need less food to feel sated. In healthy people, portion control is the result of fulfillment from food. Really. You eat less when it tastes better. Does higher quality food mean we need to shop at high-end stores and buy expensive items? Of course not. In fact, as we buy fresh, seasonal, and unprocessed items, we usually spend less per ounce than frozen pre-prepped entrees or deli take out.

Mediterranean Diet

(Once again I use the term "diet" to describe the typical foods consumed in a particular region, not a restrictive program.)

Surrounding the azure Mediterranean Sea are millions of healthy, trim people. Yet, these regions of the world are renowned for their toothsome, buttery-rich food. How is this the case? Why are the people of Italy, Greece, Southern France, and the Baltics not dropping like flies from obesity, diabetes, and heart disease? Along with a more active lifestyle, the explanation may lie in their lack of processed food and their regular intake of super foods cultivated in their region. These Mediterranean super foods include: tomatoes, lemons, garlic, olive oil, grapes, herbs, fish, grains, leafy greens like spinach, mushrooms, avocados, berries, melons, pomegranates, and figs. These are all packed with nutrition, omega 3 fatty-acids, and antioxidants, and they are consumed daily in that area of the world. To incorporate these power-foods into your day, try a squeeze of lemon in your water, fresh cut tomato on your salad, a drizzle of olive oil on your pasta, a handful of spinach alongside your fish, and a piece of fresh seasonal fruit. Try a shot of grape juice at dinner for a heart-healthy boost. Grapes don't need to ferment in barrels to provide the cholesterol lowering and antioxidant benefits touted in the media. In fact, fresh grapes provide a healthier option than wine. A little bit of these items goes a long way toward daily health.

Treats

Treat time is the unequaled, best part of my day—the moment when my body asks me for some chocolate or a cinnamon graham cracker or a lemon biscotti…you get the picture. It happens around 3:00 p.m., after I have work and family under control, and just before the kids come home.

From 3:00 p.m. – 4:00 p.m., there is a magical vacuum of quiet peace in my day. This is when my body asks for a treat. Only the best will do because, doggone it, I need a little happy to get me through the rest of the day. Prompts for a treat are not the same thing as triggers. Because fuel and pleasure are legitimate reasons for eating, those moments of pure pleasure are a welcome bit of fun in the day. On the other hand, triggers spawn unhealthy reasons for eating—like escape. As long as I tune in to my prompt and enjoy an *appropriate* treat, I perpetuate a healthy mindset. To make sure the treat is appropriate, I consider what I have already eaten today and listen to my body. Some days I feel like a piece a fruit dipped in chocolate ganache (equal parts chocolate melted with cream). Other days, a straightforward oatmeal cookie will do nicely. A nice square of dark chocolate is another of my favorites. A spoonful of peanut butter (made from 100% peanuts) swirled into a spoonful of chocolate ice cream is another home run. If I happen to have a piece of Key lime tart on hand, well, it would just be wrong to let it sit untouched in the fridge. Don't you think?

Use wisdom. Choose high-quality treats without hydrogenated fats. Portion out a small amount of huge flavor. Enjoy every bite and don't take more bites than you need. If you can, bake your own cookies, cupcakes, or brownies and keep them frozen in a re-sealable bag. Recognize the urge for a treat and satisfy it, using the principle of compensation judiciously. If I choose raspberries drizzled with chocolate syrup for my afternoon treat (because they are low in sugar and fat), I can still have corn on the cob at dinner. However, after a big Almond

Brownie (see recipes), I will choose fewer carbs at dinner, perhaps taking a pass on the bread and spooning up a little less rice.

TIP 19

Go to Bed Empty & Sleep 7-10 Hours

Go to Bed Empty & Sleep

As a general rule, go to bed empty, not hungry, and you will wake up lighter. Arrange your life so you can eat dinner early. This allows you to go to bed at a reasonable time. Eating dinner after 8:00 p.m. not only means you are starving by the time you get that meal—so you eat more than you should—but it also means you are still full at bedtime. An engorged tummy makes it difficult to sleep and can push your bedtime later than you want. Studies show people who sleep 7-9 hours a night are significantly less likely to be overweight than those who do not (*Hellmich, 8*). Turns out we have two critical appetite hormones. One called Ghrelin makes us hungry while the other one, Leptin, makes us feel full. Guess which one is produced when we are tired? Naturally, the hungry hormone—and so we eat more when we are tired. The full hormone goes on vacation when we are under-slept, which is not helpful at all (*Mignot, 3*). Being tired also induces impulse eating because our body signals don't communicate properly—we can't tell what the body is saying when we are numb from exhaustion. In hope of an energy boost, we tend to eat food high in sugars or fats when our bodies just need sleep. This puts us out of balance.

Hunger is no fun. It is uncomfortable and not to be ignored. If you find you are hungry at bedtime, have something small that fulfills what your body asks for—like a graham cracker and warm milk. Going to bed early also eliminates the possibility of late-night fridge raiding. If you struggle with nighttime cravings, go to bed before they hit. Over time, going to bed an hour earlier could reduce your daily intake of food by several hundred calories, adding up to pretty consistent weight loss and changing a lifelong habit of late-night bingeing.

The Perfect Machine

The human body is the greatest machine ever created. In Chapter 5, under *Mortal Bodies*, I compare our bodies to a sacred temple. Caring for a temple requires a different level of commitment than managing a run-down garden shed. But, from a scientific standpoint, the body is even more spectacular than any grand building. The body is greater than any machine ever invented. Our brains are the models for computers. Early computer programmers relied on known logic pathways to make programs more user friendly. Even today, the process of reverse brain engineering, which analyzes how the brain works in order to figure out how to duplicate its function in machines, is resulting in breathtaking advances in computation that will pave the way for faster, more powerful computers (*Kurzweil, 73, 117, 120, 122, 143-203*). Pioneers of the artificial heart drew their inspiration from our actual hearts—an organ so strong, sensitive, and long-lasting that with all our technology and brilliance, we can barely approximate its effectiveness. A myriad of other technologies and inventions that change the world are based on a template of the very systems we take for granted every time we take a breath, blink our eyes, or laugh. We occupy incredible machines and yet we often forget to care for them as such.

Like a Ferrari™, if we don't take the body out for a spin regularly and carefully, it will cease to perform well. A high-performance engine needs to be run. So do we. It needs great fuel and regular maintenance. So do we. Remember, if we don't use it, we lose it. I see my body with the awe and appreciation afforded a sexy sports car—it is the perfect machine.

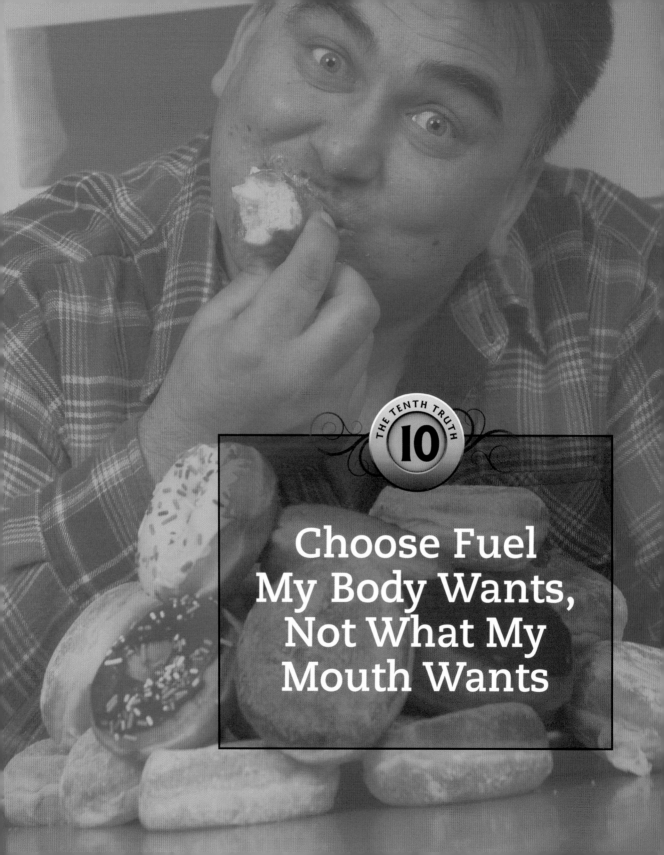

THE TENTH TRUTH

10

Choose Fuel My Body Wants, Not What My Mouth Wants

What is the difference between the desires of my body and the cravings of my mouth? My body wants the food that will make it feel well, balanced, and energetic. The mouth just wants taste, with no regard to how you will feel later. Sometimes the mouth doesn't even care about taste, it just wants to chew. Decide to make menu choices on behalf of your body, rather than from the standpoint of strictly how something tastes in your mouth. This is a different way of deciding what to eat. Instead of thinking solely about the creamy taste of beef stroganoff with noodles, envision how your whole self will feel immediately after eating it, or twenty minutes later, or an hour later. If you are skiing on a cold winter day, the stroganoff may be exactly what you need. However, if your body tells you it will feel heavy, greasy, and saturated, consider choosing a turkey sandwich instead. Your body should have a voice in the matter don't you think? Stop taking orders from your mouth. Having said that, when you really need a bagel with cream cheese, eat the bagel and compensate after.

How does listening to my body change my choices? Even when I travel or eat at a buffet restaurant, I consider first what my body wants, not what my mouth wants. If I need a grilled chicken breast and broccoli, I will go to great lengths to satisfy my body's request or get as close to it as possible. Maybe the restaurant doesn't have broccoli, but they probably have a salad or other green vegetable option. I know I will feel vigorous after a sushi meal as opposed to fried chicken with mashed potatoes which will wipe me out for hours.

If you can project zero net effect from a caramel apple, enjoy. As you eat it, pay attention to the signals you get from your body—it might surprise you. Suppose after three bites you feel sugared out and your body tells you it's had enough of the cloyingly sweet caramel. Normally, you might ignore the message and keep eating because caramel is sweet and sweet is good, right? Well, no. There is a point where you hit your sugar limit. When you start listening to your body, sweet does not taste good beyond your limit; your brain is telling you it doesn't need it. Respond to the message and stop. Wrap it up for later, give it away, or throw it away (because waste is okay)—but stop eating it.

If it sounds like you will never again eat meatloaf, think again. Our lives are so filled with special occasions, holidays, celebrations, business events, impromptu treats, and family get-togethers that it can be difficult to find time to *sandwich* in some quality choices (groan!). Healthy people choose food their body needs with enough regularity that when the pork roast dinner is served by Aunt Petunia, it can be graciously enjoyed without too much impact.

As you choose what your body wants instead of what your mouth wants you will discover how delicious real food tastes. Like cool water on a parched tongue, nothing tastes as good as the thing your body needs most. When you need asparagus and you eat fresh, tender stalks steamed to perfect tenderness, drizzled with extra-virgin olive oil, the asparagus truly satisfies more than a greasy corn dog. Trust yourself. Listen to your body and predict the impact of your choices.

The World in a Day

Every day should contain all the elements of health and balance as requested by your body. Each day we will need lots of water, the complex carbohydrates and bran found in whole grains, vegetables and fruits, some protein, dairy, and treats. Fats are already present in our sauces, meat, cheese and dairy products, and of course, in our treats. Sounds simple enough, but when you record your food choices in the following food journal, it may reveal some surprising trends. Do you really get enough water? Does the bulk of your meals come from vegetables and whole grains? Do you have a high-quality treat every day? Focus on today and don't worry about tomorrow. Make today a completely balanced day by fulfilling all your body's needs as illustrated in the following graphic.

THE WORLD
IN A DAY

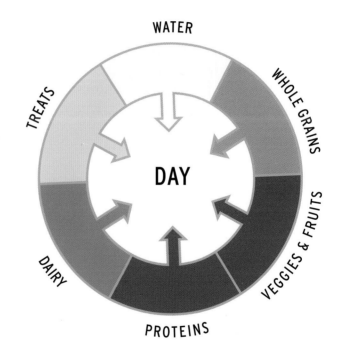

Food Journal Exercise

Although I don't subscribe to many regimens, keeping a food journal (for 2 days) is useful in this instance. It shows where your nutritional gaps may be and lets you know how to fill them. Use the following pages to map just two days of eating. Record everything you eat below the appropriate heading. For instance, I have recorded, in the following sample lunch menu the elements of my turkey sandwich on whole wheat bread, an orange, and a cookie. I listed 2 slices of bread under whole grain, 2 slices of turkey under protein, a glob of mayonnaise under oils, lettuce and tomato under vegetables, an orange under fruit, and a cookie in the treats category. Pretty basic.

Rather than include elaborate tables of how much bread equals a single serving and how much mayonnaise equals a "glob," I intentionally leave the determination of portions up to you, the reader. Whether a "glob" is the equivalent of one tablespoon or two tablespoons is not as important as adjusting the size of your "glob" to meet the needs of your metabolism. If you need more fat that day, increase your "glob"—if you need less fat, decrease it. Two ounces of turkey may be just enough for a petite woman, whereas six ounces may be just right for a man. Some days, I need two slices of thick bread on my sandwich, and other days, I take only one thin slice for an open face sandwich. The point is not to count calories, use measuring spoons, or live with rigid rules. The point is to habitually adjust portion size for your needs that day.

SAMPLE LUNCH ENTRY									
Veg	Whole Grains	White Flour	Proteins	Fruit	Dairy	Water	Oil & Fat	Treats	Sugar
Lettuce, Tomato	2 slices		2 slices turkey	1 orange			Glob mayo	1 cookie	

After you complete the journal, examine the results. Do you ingest more meat and refined white flour than vegetables and whole grain? Are there more sugars and fats on the menu than your body needs? Try to broaden your daily choices so you enjoy the *World in a Day* as illustrated on the previous page.

FOOD JOURNAL DAY #1									
Veg	Whole Grains	White Flour	Proteins	Fruit	Dairy	Water	Oil & Fat	Treats	Sugar

FOOD JOURNAL DAY #2									
Veg	Whole Grains	White Flour	Proteins	Fruit	Dairy	Water	Oil & Fat	Treats	Sugar

Compensate Meal-to-Meal

I know we have covered compensation before, but I am bringing it up again because it directly relates to the results of the journal exercise above. Inspect your entries to determine imbalances in your diet and when you next get hungry, ask yourself, *"What have I already eaten today and what do I still need?"* Based on the answer, select your meal or snack. When the PTA meeting busts out doughnuts right around lunchtime (and you are famished), you may decide to have one. This is where the law of compensation comes in: after the doughnut have a light lunch and for your afternoon treat something healthy, like a few grapes and a cup of herb tea. At dinner, you might take fewer raviolis and fill up on the salad, veggies, and strawberries. Compensate meal to meal and the doughnut will have no effect on your waistline. Don't get fancy counting fat grams or measuring salad dressing. Just be aware of what and how much your body needs to burn fat as fuel and compensate accordingly.

As you grow accustomed to adjusting your intake based on previous meals, you will become fully aware of bloated-ness, heaviness, or any kind of excess. Eventually, you will gage your meal choices on how you feel as much as on what you last ate. If you want to know what "saturated and heavy" feels like, listen to your body after you have had too much lasagna with sausage. On the other hand, nobody ever felt saturated after 2 days of salad. The difference between choosing what your mouth wants verses what your body wants is a light, energized, clean feeling, as opposed to feeling saturated.

Compensate Day-to-day

Compensate on a daily basis. Some overloads require several meals of compensation to negate the effects. My day after Christmas includes low salt, vegetables, little protein, minimal starch, and small portions. I will enjoy maybe one leftover Christmas cookie, but if your holiday dinner is like mine, you will want to compensate by NOT finishing the tin of toffees.

Compensate Week-to-week

Because some overindulgent events go on for days, we may need to compensate for weeks. Plan ahead for holidays and travel—eat lean before you go. Having said that, if you end up noshing your way through Italy for ten days, apply the law of compensation for several weeks, after you arrive home, until your system sheds those pasta pounds and your bowels regulate.

Compounding the Excess

Beware of chasing a week of heavy meals with more heavy meals. For instance, let's say you go on a cruise, knowing in advance it will involve a lot of food. You can allow some indulgence, because as my brother always says, *"When you go on vacation, don't stay home."* But, after stuffing yourself for a week, do not come home and continue to over-eat the wrong food. It is easy to do. We tend to stick our proverbial fingers in our ears and tell our bodies, *"I'm not listening; I'm not listening…."*. If we override those little cues for salad long enough, the body stops sending them. Suddenly, our cruise shorts don't even button anymore. We can blame the cruise, but the lovely cruise staff did not follow us home and continue to force feed us. We really gained twenty pounds from refusing to listen to our bodies *after* the vacation. The damage from the vacation could have been easily shed in a few weeks by compensating.

Daily Timing

Timing counts. We must eat to keep our metabolisms fast, but to lose excess weight, we must expend more fuel than we take in. Here are some important behaviors:

• Start the day with minimal fat—fat in the morning makes us crave it all day long

• Keep protein in diet mid-day

• Snack in afternoon so you don't overeat at dinner—lots of flavor, small quantities

• Enjoy a small dinner built around vegetables, grains, and lean proteins

• Go to bed empty (not hungry)

• Have a fall back plan for the nighttime munchies (such as Pero®, herb tea, berries, watermelon, bitter chocolate (dark), almonds, graham crackers and milk, etc.)—and see the following after-dinner coping strategies, along with Tip #21 on page 144.

TIP 20

Eating Fat Makes Me Want More Fat Our tastes tend to run with what we usually eat. If I eat a lot of hamburger, I will continue to crave saturated fat. If I eat a lot of tortilla chips, I will crave oil and salt. Soda makes me want more soda. It only takes a few days of eating healthy to crave more healthy food because our mouths want more of the same.

Strategies

The following strategies help keep your body balanced and revving at full throttle during real-life situations. I like to call these strategies: *know before you go.*

Restaurants

When you go out to eat, plan on choosing what your body wants regardless of the other menu choices. Ask for half portions. Unless you "hork" down your food you will probably be full by the time you finish the salad course anyway so it just saves money to get a half portion. If you order your dressings and sauces on the side, you are more likely to get the nod from your bod to enjoy a few bites of dessert. Drink water—it doesn't cost a dime and you can't get drunk or fat from water. Besides, you need it. If your body wants bread, enjoy it, but don't let the social atmosphere lull you into a false sense of escape. One roll is enough. White bread turns to sugar which most assuredly turns into fat. Think of your dining choices as not about limiting yourself, but as thoughtful decisions made from hearing the needs of your fantastic body.

Holidays

It takes most of us nine months to undo the damage we do in two months over the holidays. Fall comes with colder weather and the nesting instinct to bundle up and eat comfort food. Add to this season a ramped-up social calendar with meals clocking in at over 5000 calories, and you have a recipe for weight gain. I like to joke that I am allergic to holiday food—it makes my thighs swell.

With so many pitfalls and tins of caramel, what can we do to keep a healthy balance and speedy metabolism? First and foremost, don't let your exercise wane. During winter weather, many walking/running programs bite the dust. Get an excellent indoor workout option, like a treadmill or a workout video. Use it when you cannot go out. Budget time so you keep exercise firmly in the schedule. Just do it. Power through.

Pay close attention to compensation during the holidays. You might encounter food obligations every day that require a bit of planning. Anticipate an upcoming party by eating light beforehand. After the event, choose whole grains, light soups, salads, and sandwiches to counteract the cheese balls and cocktail weenies.

Another aspect of holiday management is to stay centered with enough sleep and personal time. Even though we do fun things during the holidays, we can get so busy we can start to feel haggard. It becomes all too easy to seek comfort in munching. Find ten minutes to walk around the block and just think. Take a bath and pet the cat (maybe not at the same time). Paint your toenails. Stop talking and turn off the television. Be with yourself. Surprisingly, quiet time alone allows you to be fed in a very real way. Keep your self-talk positive and affirming.

Be aware of triggers. In anticipation of the in-laws, don't try and hide in the clam dip. Express your anxieties out loud, preferably when you are out of earshot of the offending party. For instance, in the privacy of your own room, say, "I am going to spend five days with my Mother-in-law. Oh snap!" Owning a potential trigger helps us see them for what they are. Most anxieties, when expressed aloud, are not monsters at all. Dread and worry don't deserve a compulsive reaction, they just need to be acknowledged as real. If you know your boss is an eating trigger, stay away from him or her at the office party. Talk to the weird receptionist, play bingo, do what you have to, but triumph over the triggers.

Obligations

Being a guest of someone else's hospitality can mean saying "yes" to food you otherwise don't need. There are times when it would be rude to refuse. For a couple of meals, I can eat whatever my hosts offer. However, for an extended period of time, it becomes necessary to graciously select what I need to feel well. This is also true of food gifts. When your boss sets a box of chocolates on your desk, for heaven's sake, have a chocolate and enjoy it (make sure he sees you eating and smiling). Then take the rest of the chocolates home and enjoy one each day until they are gone. Why not? Your daily routine includes a treat. Compensation is the key.

Availability

Sometimes you just cannot get what your body needs. I spent 5 days in Austria with nary a vegetable in sight. I can only eat pork products for so long. When I asked for vegetables, I got a potato. Nonetheless, I did the best I could. I took a daily walk through the Salzburg outdoor market, chomping on raw carrots and turnips. When light food is not available, choose whole grains instead of white flour. Keep with lean meat and fish, continuing to drink lots of water helps, and limiting pastries and sweets helps. And when you again get to eat simple meals with vegetables, use the law of compensation to recover.

No Time

When there is no time to sit down and really taste food, we can all too easily get in the habit of scarfing down our meals. Not tasting means not feeling satisfied. Eating fast can result in eating too much and choosing the wrong food for your metabolism. When pressed for time, we have to get whatever is available and therein lies our all-too busy dilemma: how do we give our bodies what they need when our plane boards in five minutes and there is no spinach salad at 30,000 feet?

> **Don't be afraid of hunger. Hunger means you have another chance to eat the fuel your body asks for.**

The prosaic answer is to do the best you can. Try to plan ahead. A peanut butter sandwich on whole wheat bread, wrapped up the night before, can stave off many a drive-thru impulse. It can keep you going until you can find a healthy option. You don't want to get so hungry you override your need for a salad bar with a paper boat of nachos. Keep emergency snacks handy like an apple, a bottle of water, and some granola bars or whole-wheat (non-hydrogenated) crackers. When you finally have access to quality food, pay attention to it. Savor the flavor, even if you can only focus while you are stopped at a red light. Remember to taste. Especially important is the need to slow down your chewing. Don't stuff. It's better to only have time to ingest a few bites of hot dog than to create the habit of wolfing down the whole tamale just because it is there. It's ok to be hungry again in a few hours. Don't be afraid of hunger. Hunger means you have another chance to eat the fuel your body asks for.

Too Hungry

Have you ever been so hungry your body becomes weak and shaky, the kind of hunger that makes you feel sick and crazy for food? This condition can make you end up shoveling in whatever you can lay your hands on before you pass out.

When you are too hungry to make a healthy meal choice, you are more likely to eat whatever is quick and within reach, like the entire bag of breakfast cereal. Try to respond to your needs before you get to this point. For instance, during long gaps between meals, dole out a handful of almonds or an orange to keep you alive while you simmer your bean stew.

We should eat every 4-5 hours, more often as your body prompts. When you are headed out the door for exercise have a swig of milk or juice before you go to keep you fueled. When you are absolutely famished, continue to listen to your body instead of your mouth. The quick option is usually not the best choice. For instance, the frozen Pasta Alfredo may only take two minutes to microwave, but the thirty-minute stir-fry vegetables with chicken might be what your body needs. Take a drink of juice or eat a slice of bread until the stir-fry is ready. Practice delaying gratification and it will become easier over time. Remember, there will always be quicker foods, but nothing tastes as good as what your body really needs.

Missed Meals

Just like the above strategies for managing a lack of time, keep healthy snacks on-hand to cope with missed meals. Also, avoid skipping meals if possible. The common sense rule is to get on a schedule. Eat at least three meals a day. Nothing makes it more difficult to calmly assess your body's needs than to be hyper-hungry. By the time 3:00 p.m. rolls around, you should not be desperate for your first meal of the day. Along the same lines, drinking a diet shake for breakfast and lunch and then pigging out all night long is not a formula for lifelong health and balance. Eat breakfast, even if it is only a nectarine and a granola bar. Eat lunch, choosing whatever your body needs. Have a snack in the afternoon and carefully choose the timing and contents of your dinner, compensating if necessary.

Late Night Parties and Treats

Akin to managing the holidays and various food obligations is handling late night parties. The midnight chocolate buffet might sound fun, but after listening to your body and getting on a healthy schedule, the timing of dessert at midnight may not work for you. Maybe you could just wrap up a piece of cake and save it in the fridge until *you* are ready for it.

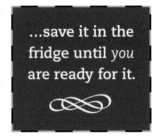

...save it in the fridge until *you* are ready for it.

Eating consistently late at night will not end well. It can be compared to the "sumo diet." Sumo training methods are reported to include withholding food during the day and then gorging at night right before going to sleep. The net effect is, apparently, huge. So, when the buttered popcorn is passed around during a late movie what do you do? Use a cup, a bag, or a napkin and take an acceptable amount of popcorn (same thing applies to candy, ice cream, nachos, etc.). Your portion might be just a few mouthfuls. Remember to focus on quality and not quantity. Keep only your chosen amount within reach; i.e. send that elephant-size popcorn bucket down the row so it does not stay in your lap. Don't use the popcorn as an escape. Eat it slowly and taste it. If any food has an off-taste or if it doesn't really satisfy, throw it away. A surprising amount of junk food has a rancid aftertaste. It is easy to detect poor quality once you get past the initial hit of sugar or salt on your tongue. After savoring each mouthful, if you still crave more popcorn, fill up on a tall glass of water with lemon to close off the taste buds. Practice this behavior and it will become a habit.

When the evening celebration concludes with a piece of wedding cake, please have some. A small slice of cake is good—one whole tier is not. Simply pick yourself up the next day and compensate with a little less bread or starch. No harm done.

Sick Days

In truth, little strategy is needed during the period of time you are off your feet, wheezing and hacking in bed—because let's face it, while feeling rotten we do what we have to do to get through it. No, it is the days and weeks following your illness that require more diligence. If, during your Kleenex-filled sabbatical you have unfortunately subscribed to the home-remedy of "eating your way through a cold", you may find your nose chapped and your jeans tighter at the end of your ordeal. Recognize that just because you cannot taste the sherbet doesn't mean it has lost its caloric value. Try not to overdo during illness, and then resume exercise and light meals as soon as possible. Compensate, compensate, compensate. Use those brothy chicken soup days to your advantage. No one ever gained weight on soup—even when consumed in a supine position with a spoon in one hand and a remote control in the other. If your affliction happened to fall into the gastro-intestinal category, just be comforted by the knowledge that, in the words of my wise mother-in-law, "Throwing up and diarrhea are good for five pounds." And, when you feel better gingerly enter back into your exercise routine because you may be weak and dehydrated.

How to Avoid Eating After Dinner

If you experience a compulsion to snack after dinner, you are pretty normal. Having said that, grazing into the night can easily undo all the balanced choices you made during the day. Here are a few tips to prevent evening escapes down the cookie trail. First, enjoy a diverse dinner with lots of colors on your plate. Deficiencies in your diet can trigger cravings. For example, a dinner made up entirely of noodles will leave you wanting the nutritional value of vegetables and protein and, consequently, you will continue to feel cravings that often take the form of junk food.

Second, plan your eating so you can digest your dinner well before bedtime. Remember Tip #19 in Chapter 9—*Go to bed empty, not hungry*. Listen to your body to determine what time you need to be in bed so you don't feel hunger, and what time you need to eat so you can be sufficiently empty. If you are eating pot roast tonight, you may need to start at 5:30 p.m. in order to be empty by 10:00 p.m. However, any of the vegetarian entrees in the recipe portion of this book will render an empty feeling within 2-3 hours of eating. If you eat a lot of salad at dinner with a small portion of meat and starch, you will be empty within only a few hours.

If you don't have the liberty of selecting an optimal time to eat, exercise portion control to offset that late dinner. Half of a serving will take half as long to digest. It also has half the dilatory affect on your metabolism which means you keep your fine machine humming at a fat-burning rate.

TIP 21

Have a Warm Drink at Night to Curb Munchies. A big mug of Pero™ instant hot beverage (a caffeine-free drink made from grain) fills my belly at night and curbs the desire to munch. I take it straight or stir in ½ -teaspoon of cocoa powder and a splash of milk to take off the bitter edge. There are many other brands of these kinds of coffee substitutes— all are good, but Pero™ and Caffix™ are widely available and both are excellent. Because barley and malt hot beverages have no caffeine, no calories, and a pleasing bitterness, they finish off my palette for the day and arrest my desire for more food.

Third, not only are hot, non-caffeinated drinks a great way to stay hydrated as mentioned in Chapter 9, but they also help prevent a nighttime binge. Keep your house stocked with soothing helpers like *Pero®* barley beverage, and herb tea. Also, bittersweet chocolate, lemons for your water, herb tea, rye crackers, and raw unsalted nuts can serve the same function. This is such a helpful technique, I included it above in *Tip #21*.

Finally, as a reminder, resist eating at night by going to sleep. Don't read. Turn off the television and go to bed. It only takes a few weeks to train your brain to sleep a little earlier than usual. Over time, sleeping instead of snacking saves you thousands of calories as it creates a healthier, permanent habit.

Conclusion

You can do all this! How do I know? Because most of the concepts you just read are things you already knew to be true. Acquiring new habits is realistic—you have assimilated new skills before, haven't you? Becoming the caretaker of your new, thin body is no different than learning a new computer program, a foreign language, new math concepts, a sequence of dance steps, or learning how to read and write.

Becoming a new person on the outside really requires two things: changing how you think on the inside and committing to the permanency of the changes. When continually applied to your daily life, the principles in these pages can actually change the way you think, in a sustainable, enjoyable way—causing your body to shed unnecessary weight.

Eat, and eat well. Live abundantly with excitement and anticipation for pleasure. Experience all the good stuff in life while at the same time enjoying a healthier body. Shake off the old mores that proscribe pleasure and fun. Trust your body. It will deliver all the messages and signals you require to maintain perfect harmony every day.

In addition, trust the designer of your body—He loves you at every stage and size. When you were in diapers, He treasured you. In adulthood, He continues to love you to an indescribable degree. And at the frail, feeble moments of old age, He holds you close with priceless tenderness. Fat or thin is not nearly so important to The Lord as *who* you become. Hopefully, you will use the time you have in life to become more like your Heavenly Father. In this context, don't betray yourself. Treat yourself with the same care and consideration you show to others, which means making your personal health paramount. Do whatever it takes to learn wise, new habits.

Be honest and vigilant about exercise—don't rationalize it away. Be patient. Great things happen one day at a time. Pursue knowledge about food and exercise. Become balanced. Most of all, treasure your soul now, as it is today, and each remaining day of your life. Be thankful for your life and your blessings. Pray in gratitude. Pray for wisdom. Pray for strength. Now, power through!

"Congratulations! Today is your day!
You're off to great places! You're off and away!"

(DR. SUESS, 1)

To remain enlightened remember these 10 Truths

1. Get the click

2. Health is beauty

3. Diets make me fat

4. Change the inside and the outside will eventually respond

5. What I think, say, and do, I become

6. Does my health program pass the test: ...'til I'm 80?

7. Consistency not intensity

8. Treat my body like a Ferrari™

9. Quality, not quantity

10. Choose fuel my body wants, not what my mouth wants

References

Troubleshooting

1   **Question:** When I try to visualize my body in its ideal form, I cannot conjure up that picture in my mind because I don't have any idea what it would look like. I feel uncomfortable trying to envision an unrealistic image. How do I fantasize about something I cannot even imagine?

Solution: Use physical activity to springboard into the following mental exercise. Attempt this visualization during exercise because your attitude will be more positive and your endorphins will be pumping.

To begin, take a moment during exercise to feel gratitude for the health and strength you feel. Say a prayer of thanks if you are inclined. Then, engage your core (abdominal muscles). Flex them until you can feel a flattening of the belly. It may not actually look flatter, but continue to contract your belly until your navel sinks toward your spine. Use good posture and stay relaxed. Breathe in a steady rhythm.

With your core engaged, envision your body as you would like it to be. Starting with your head and shoulders, elongate your neck, imagining it long and lean. Continue picturing your shoulders with well-formed tone. See your chest as firm and strong. Keep breathing. Picture your back with supple muscles cinching in at the waist. Proceed down to your belly, hips and legs. Take a step and actually feel in your stride how you would walk if your thighs no longer brushed together. Imagine the amount of impact your knees and feet would support at your ideal weight. How would your joints feel? Be light and buoyant as you do this exercise.

Now fix in your mind an overall view of your ideal self from the inside out. With kindness tell yourself, *"This is me, who I really am."* Accept your ideal self.

Do this every day for maximum benefit.

2   **Question:** What if I feel much thinner than I really am? I look in the mirror and become dejected by what I see.

Solution: Good for you for feeling trim. It is easier to perform effective visualization when you already have a healthy mental picture of yourself and don't need to overcome a negative body image. Apply all *10 Truths* to your life to re-connect with your body's messages until your behaviors mimic those of a thin person. Be consistent and patient. With time your body will ultimately match the image in your head.

3 **Question:** I don't hear my body asking for anything in particular. I am just hungry. Lots of different things sound good and I am not sure which to choose. What should I eat?

Solution: The goal is to connect your desire for food with your body's needs. Begin by forming an image in your mind of high-value foods. Which foods? Let's start with the foods that fuel your metabolism—like vegetables and whole grains. Picture a crisp green salad with colorful vegetables and your favorite salad dressing. Now imagine a fluffy pilaf of brown rice with pesto, walnuts, and dried cranberries. If the salad and pilaf sound good, you probably need them. Try to eat them or something comparable at your next meal.

Keep dreaming about a mélange of foods, and decide what other vegetables tickle your taste buds? If red radishes, sweet yellow bell peppers, and green zucchini stand out, add them to your salad. Do you want mushrooms, sprouts, and broccoli? Tune in to flashes of interest and go shopping. As you peruse the produce in the market, if any fruits and vegetables look good to you, take them home because your body is trying to tell you they contain nutrients you need today. Fulfilling requests encourages your body to tell you what it needs.

Now, consider adding some protein to your salad. Does fish or chicken sound good? Tuna fish tastes great atop salad. Would you enjoy a little bread dipped in olive oil and balsamic vinegar? Go ahead, bon appétit. Select only 100% whole grain bread—I like the crusty kind. Choose the bread amount that is right for you today. Have a large glass of water with your salad, tuna, and bread. (All of these things can be ordered at most restaurants.)

For ease, wash and cut up raw vegetables and fruits so they are readily available during the week. They store well in a re-closeable freezer bag. Taste them just as you would chocolate to evaluate quality. Keep extra servings of steamed brown rice, barley, or quinoa in the fridge to pile on top of your salad or to enjoy alongside your protein—such as shrimp with leeks and zucchini.

Purchase seasonal fresh fruit and vegetables, whenever possible, because they taste better. Buy the highest quality you can afford. Organic is great, but it is not essential.

When it's time for your next meal, repeat this process: think about whole grains, fruit, vegetables, fish and lean proteins. Fulfill your hunger with the foods that sound appealing. Round out your meal with other food groups to create balance. Add a handful of strawberries and a slice of baked yam—the more colors on your plate, the better. Notice which foods taste good *and* make you feel energetic. A lot of foods taste good in the mouth, but don't provide vigor and strength to the body. Allow your body to help choose your food. As you picture healthy food choices and respond to the ones your body wants, you will be encouraging your body to give you more signals

4 **Question:** Whenever I start choosing good food and I start losing weight, I self-sabotage with binge eating. How do I stay on track?

Answer: Do these four things: re-set your baseline to a more moderate expectation of exercise (no pain), become fearless about change, resist wallowing in useless guilt, and love yourself. Remember, weight loss is a consequence of staying on track. Even so, getting off track is normal. Getting back on track is priceless. The trick lies in reformatting your thoughts and emotions to aide, not hinder, healthy habits, which is the miracle in the *10 Truths*.

As you become healthier, the result will likely be weight loss, which, surprisingly, makes many people nervous. A typical nervous response is ramping up your exercise baseline to a non-sustainable level of intensity—which results in abandoning your exercise after a short while. Also typical are feelings of anxiety. Anxiety over losing weight is normal. It manifests as compulsions and cravings—which can make you want to EAT!

Taking care of our bodies requires love. It takes courage to throw off the shackles and lies that keep us trapped in unhealthy thoughts and behaviors. If you feel resistant to these changes, remember *your choice* to be balanced and healthy. You have decided to feel comfortable in your own skin. Keep your baseline moderate and bravely face the changes in your life as your body changes.

5 **Question:** I am frustrated. I have followed all *10 Truths* in this book for over a month, but nothing has happened. The scale says I weigh the same as I did when I started. I exercise six days a week and eat balanced portions of healthy food. Am I the exception to the rule? Are there people that regularly make healthy choices, yet they don't lose fat? If I don't see any results, why should I keep trying?

Answer: The hardest thing to sell is patience. But, tenacity is exactly what you need. Let's compare your situation to mowing the lawn which, for the purposes of this analogy, let us say, you hate doing. You can plant, over time, a slow-growing variety of grass that never again needs mowing. This new variety is more desirable, but it will take a fair amount of cultivating to take hold. Daily watering and weeding is required. It might take months. However, once established, it only requires easy upkeep to maintain. Or, you can continue to mow the old grass knowing full well it will need to be mowed again next week. Nothing changes permanently with the old grass—it just equals more confounded mowing. New grass requires time, but it changes the way you live because it is prettier and it requires less mowing (and now your Saturdays are free).

These *10 Truths* are the new variety of grass. The new grass gives you what you really want. Diets and weight-loss programs are like mowing the old variety of lawn over and over.

Stepping away from yard-work, let's return to the question: "Am I the exception to the rule?" Rest assured your body *will* transform. It takes time for your brain to get the message to use fat for fuel. The longer you have been storing fat (instead of using it for energy), the more time it will take to release it. Eventually, your thighs will get with the program and take on a lean shape commensurate with the activity in your life. In the meantime, you will benefit while you wait. Every good choice you make today reinforces the likelihood you will make a good choice again tomorrow—thus building healthy habits. As you consistently behave like a trim person, you will become that person. Every body responds this way and yours will, too.

May I please remind you I waited six months for my body to respond to these new habits? It may not take that long, or it could take longer—but your body will respond.

Check to make sure your regular intake of grains come from whole grain, and avoid hydrogenated fat and high-fructose corn syrup. We sometimes overlook the large part these play in "regular food." Something so easy as switching to whole wheat bread will, over time, accelerate your weight loss.

Diet products and programs make millions of dollars because they promise speedy results. Like mowing the lawn, they take your money over and over again. Remember, diets are designed to be fleeting and cause you to repeatedly need their products. You already know this is true. Don't cave in to impatience and falsehoods. There is no short-cut to lifelong weight control except to embody lifelong weight control. Start today and only worry about today. Don't get overwhelmed worrying about tomorrow or the next day. Find ways to be healthier today than you were yesterday. Be positive and grateful for your body and mind. Fill your spirit with uplifting things. Be happy and your body will respond when it is ready.

Sample Menus

Although the most important message of this book is to listen to your individual needs and respond to them, many people have asked me what a typical day looks like in terms of food. What is a balanced day? In response, I have created the following sample menus to illustrate what my particular body might ask for in a typical day. Your needs may be different. Your metabolism and activity level may be different. Your tastes probably differ from mine. Some people find they eat too much protein, but otherwise have a pretty good handle on their diet. Others load excess carbohydrates into their systems at night. Use the food journals in chapter 10 to identify habits that keep you out of balance. Small adjustments repeated over time can yield huge results.

Day 1

Breakfast

> 1 cup of herb tea
> 1 cup whole grain breakfast cereal (low sugar—like wheat squares or *Cheerios*™) mixed with ½ cup homemade granola with nuts (recipe section) and enough 1% milk to cover

Mid Morning Snack

> 1 ripe nectarine
> 1 tall glass of water

Lunch

> turkey sandwich— 2 slices whole wheat bread
>   2 slices deli turkey
>   2 big squirts real mayonnaise
>   1 big dollop Dijon mustard
>   lettuce piled high
>   ½ small tomato sliced
>   ¼ sliced avocado
> tall glass of water
> handful of green grapes

Mid Afternoon Snack

1 homemade chocolate chip cookie (see recipe section)
1 tall glass of water

Dinner

5-ounces oven roasted teriyaki-glazed salmon (see recipe section)
1 cup steamed broccoli drizzled with olive oil
¾ cup brown rice with a dab of butter
dinner salad with cucumber, avocado, and radish slices
two big dollops homemade buttermilk ranch dressing (see recipes)
½ kiwi
1 tall glass of water

Bedtime Snack

1 large mug of steaming hot Caffix® with ½ teaspoon organic cocoa, stirred with a
   splash of cream and a shot of milk.
Good night.
Note: After Day #1, my body might need a little more protein, so Day #2 might look
like this:

Day 2

Breakfast

2 eggs, fried in a bit of butter and olive oil
1 slice whole-wheat toast with butter and jam
4-5 large strawberries
1 tall glass 1% milk
(No mid morning snack needed after this breakfast)

Lunch

Tuna Salad—   mixed greens
               assorted fresh vegetables
               2 big scoops tuna fish mixed with real mayo and chopped celery
                       ½ medium tomato cut up
                       ½ carrot, sliced
                       drizzle of olive oil
                       squeeze of lemon

Mid Afternoon Snack

2 small squares bittersweet chocolate
1 tall glass water

Dinner

Vegetarian white bean stew with sage (see recipes)
1 slice whole-wheat toast with butter
1 orange
1 tall glass water

Bedtime Snack

1 cup peach herb tea
1 almond biscotti cookie
Good night.

Kitchen Food Stocks

The following is a suggested list of items to keep stocked in your refrigerator, freezer, and pantry. Keeping these items on hand allows you to service your body with the foods you need. Most of these items are available in your grocery store, in the bulk food bins at a health-food store, in member warehouse clubs, or in an Asian market. Use the internet to source items not sold nearby.

Pantry Stocks

- Barley
- Oats
- Brown rice
- Basmati or jasmine white rice
- Whole-wheat couscous
- Quinoa
- Pasta—buy imported from Italy, it is far superior in texture to domestic brands
- Whole-wheat flour
- Unbleached white flour
- Corn meal
- Baking soda
- Baking powder
- Cocoa
- Semi-sweet chocolate chips—use only good quality with no added hydrogenated fats
- Powdered milk
- Sugar
- Brown sugar
- Honey
- Pure maple syrup
- Jam—assorted flavors
- Yeast
- Whole grain breakfast cereal
- Dried fruits—raisin, kiwi, mango, cranberry, prune, cherry, coconut, apple, pear, etc.
- Canned assorted beans—garbanzo, kidney, black, butter, pinto, great northern, etc.
- Canned corn
- Canned green beans
- Canned chicken stock—low sodium
- Canned beef stock
- Fish or shrimp flavored bouillon cubes
- Canned tomatoes—diced
- Canned chicken meat
- Canned tuna fish
- Olive oil
- Canola oil
- Dried chilies
- Dried herbs and spices
- Dried shitake mushrooms

Refrigerator Stocks

- Eggs
- Butter
- Milk
- Plain yogurt—I prefer whole milk yogurt
- Sour cream—full fat or reduced fat
- Parmesan cheese or other nutty-flavored, hard grating cheese like Asiago or Romano
- Buttermilk (or add lemon juice to milk as a substitute for buttermilk)
- Cream—just a half-pint comes in handy
- Fresh garlic
- Fresh ginger
- Capers
- Lemons
- Limes
- Sweet onions
- Carrots
- Celery
- Potatoes
- Green onions (scallions)
- Jalapeño peppers or other chilies—anaheim, pasilla, serrano, etc.
- Tomatoes
- Avocado—yes, after ripening they refrigerate well
- Lettuce
- Spinach
- Bottled roasted red pepper packed in brine
- Soy sauce—low sodium
- Oyster sauce
- Hoisin sauce
- Fish sauce—a Thai product found in Asian markets and some supermarkets
- Sun-dried tomatoes packed in oil
- Oranges
- Apples
- Bananas
- Fresh seasonal fruit
- Fresh seasonal vegetables
- Sliced deli turkey
- Tofu
- Dijon mustard
- Assorted nuts and seeds (keep these in the refrigerator to prevent the oils from turning rancid)

Refrigerator or Freezer

- Chicken
- Fish
- Shrimp
- Turkey breast
- Ground turkey
- Peanut Butter
- Raviolis & tortellini
- Butter—yes, it freezes well
- Peas
- Green beans
- Corn
- Bananas—to throw in a quick smoothie
- Berries

Works Cited and Referenced

Brotman, Juliano, and Erica Lenkert. *Raw: the Uncook Book*. New York: ReganBooks, 1999.

Cauter, Eve Van PhD., Tasali Spiegel, and Penev. "Brief Communication: Sleep Curtailment in Healthy Young Men is Associated with Decreased Leptin Levels, Elevated Ghrelin Levels, and Increased Hunger and Appetite." *Annals of Internal Medicine* 141.11 (2004): 846-850.

Christian, Janet L., and Janet L. Greger. *Nutrition for Living*. 2nd ed. Menlo Park: Benjamin/Cummings Publishing, 1985.

Colicos, Michael A. "Remodeling of Synaptic Action Induced by Photoconductive Stimulation." *Cell* 30 Nov. 2001: 605-16.

Cunningham, Marion. *The Fannie Farmer Cookbook*. New York: Knopf, 1990.

---. *The Fannie Farmer Baking Book*. New York: Knopf, 1984.

Hellmich, Nanci. "Sleep Loss May Equal Weight Gain." *USA Today* 8 Dec. 2004: 8.

Henderson, Marguerite Marceau. *Savor the Memories*. Nashville: Favorite Recipes Press, 2002.

Isaac, A. R. "Mental Practice—Does it Work in the Field?" *The Sport Psychologist* 6 (1992): 192-198.

Kurzweil, Ray. *The Singularity Is Near*. New York: Viking Penguin, 2005.

Martin, K.A., and C.R. Hall. "Using Mental Imagery to Enhance Intrinsic Motivation." *Journal of Sport and Exercise Psychology* 17 (1995): 1, 54-69.

Mignot, Emmanual. "Short Sleep Duration is Associated with Reduced Leptin, Elevated Ghrelin, and Increased Body Mass Index." *Public Library of Science Medicine* 1.3 (2004): 1, 8-11.

Pascual-Leone, Alvaro. "The Brain That Plays Music and Is Changed by It." *Annals of the NewYork Academy of Sciences* 930 (2001): 315-329.

Rombauer, Irma S., and Marion Rombauer. *The Joy of Cooking*. New York: Signet Books, 2001.

Shannon, Nomi. *The Raw Gourmet*. Burnaby BC, Canada: Alive Books, 1999.

Sherrid, Pamela. "Piling On the Profit." *US News & World Reports Online* 8 June, 2003: Money & Business. 5 October, 2009 <http://health.usnews.com/usnews/health/articles/030616/16profit.htm>

"Suess, Dr." Geisel Page. *Oh, The Places You'll Go*. New York: Random House, 1990: 1.

---. *Green Eggs and Ham*. New York: Random House, 1960: 53.

Tallal, Paula. "Language Comprehension in Language-Learning Impaired Children Improved with Acoustically Modified Speech." *Science* 5 Jan. 1996: 81-84.

"*The Princess Bride*." Prod. Norman Lear. Twentieth Century Fox, MGM/UA Home Entertainment, 1987.

Wolke, Robert L. *What Einstein Told His Cook*. New York: W. W. Norton & Company, Inc., 2002.

---. *What Einstein Told His Cook 2*. New York: W.W. Norton & Company, Inc., 2005.

Internet Sites & Magazines

www.Weightlossforall.com/carbohydrates.htm

www.Weightlossforall.com/fat.htm

www.Epicurious.com

www.Americanheart.org (American Heart Association)

www.Hearthighway.org/guidelines

www.Health.utah.gov/html/healthy_lifestyles (Utah Department of Health)

www.Essortment.com

www.Cheftalk.com

www.Youtube.com

Trademark Acknowledgements

All trademarks in this book are owned by the parties indicated. No ownership by the author or publisher is claimed or implied by any reference to trademarked property herein. All trademark ownership information is based on patent trademark office public registrant and owner information as of June 22, 2009.

BMW™	Registrant:	Bayerische Mortoren Werke Germany
Cafix™	Registrant/owner:	Quieta-Werke GMBH Germany
	Last listed owner:	World Finer Foods, Inc. Corporation Delaware
Cheerios™	Owner/registrant:	General Mills IP Holdings I, LLC LTD LIAB Co Delaware
Diet Coke™	Owner/applicant:	The Coca-Cola Company Corporation Delaware
Ferrari™	Owner/applicant:	Ferrari S.P.A. Unknown
Frisbee™	Owner/applicant:	Wham-O, Inc. Corporation Delaware
Fritos™	Owner/applicant:	Frito-Lay North America, Inc. Corporation Delaware

Herbalife™	Owner/registrant:	Herbalife International, Inc.
		Corporation Nevada
Hostess™	Owner/registrant:	Interstate Bakeries Corp
		Corporation Delaware
Hot Pockets™	Owner:	Chef America, Inc.
		Corporation California
	Last Listed Owner:	Societe Des Produits Nestle, S.A.
		Corporation Switzerland
Ironman™	Owner/registrant:	World Triathlon Corp
		Corporation Florida
Jenny Craig™	Owner/registrant:	Jenny Craig, Inc.
		Corporation Delaware
	Last Listed Owner:	Societe Des Produits Nestle, S.A.
		Corporation Switzerland
Keebler™	Owner/registrant:	Keebler Company
		Corporation Delaware
Kool-Aid™	Owner/registrant:	Kraft Foods, Inc.
		Corporation Delaware
	Last Listed Owner:	Kraft Foods Global Brands LLC
M&M's™	Owner/registrant:	Mars, Incorporated
		Corporation Delaware
Nutrisystem™	Owner/registrant:	Nutri/System IPHC, Inc.
		Corporation Delaware
Pero™	Registrant/owner:	Franck und Kathreiner G.M.B.H.
		Germany
	Last listed owner:	Societe Des Produits Nesle S.A.
		Corporation Assignee of Switzerland
Pharmanex™	Owner/registrant:	Pharmanex, Inc.
		Corporation Delaware
	Last listed owner:	NSE Products, Inc.
		Corporation Delaware
Slim-Fast™	Owner/registrant:	Lipton Investments, Inc.
		Corporation Delaware
	Last listed owner:	Unilever Supply Chain, Inc.
		Corporation Delaware
The Grapefruit Diet	Owner/registrant:	Omni Nutraceuticals, Inc.
		Corporation California
Twinkies™	Last listed owner:	Interstate Bakeries Corporation
		Corporation Delaware
WeightWatchers™	Owner/registrant:	Weight Watchers International, Inc.
		Corporation Virginia

Real Food
Recipes

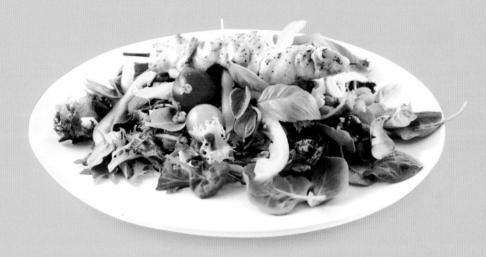

KEY

	Daily Fuel — This designation is quite arbitrary. But, in general, "daily fuel" recipes contain copious amounts of fruit, vegetables, or whole grains with minimal amounts of animal fats and sugar. These foods can be enjoyed on a daily basis or back-to-back without the need for recovery.
	Occasional Treat — consumed judiciously, only as your body indicates.
	Quickly Prepared — start-to-finish in under 30 minutes.
	Inexpensive — requires inexpensive ingredients or can be made with on-hand items listed in the pantry stock section of this book.
	Kid-Friendly and grown-up approved — not too weird, but still good.
	Vegetarian — does not contain meat, however it may contain eggs and/or dairy.
	Vegetarian-modified — contains meat, but easily modified to be meatless and/or vegan.

Breakfast

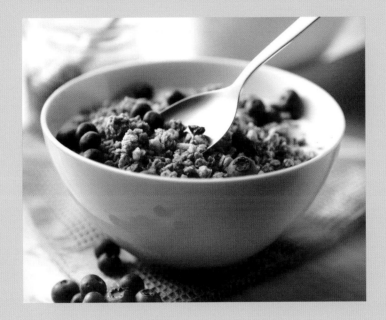

Tammy's Granola, page 166

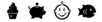

Smoked Turkey & Sweet Potato Hash with Eggs

Serves 4 as an entree

Do you remember when making fried potato hash took forever to cook? Who has time in the morning to stir potatoes for hours! The beauty of this dish is pre-cooking the 'taters (which can be done a day ahead), so browning the hash really only takes a few minutes. To avoid a mashed effect, gently toss the cooked meat with the fried potatoes before cracking the eggs over the top.

Vegetarian Modification—substitute browned tofu for the turkey or omit the turkey entirely.

You will need two very large lidded sauté (frying) pans.

3   tablespoons butter, bacon drippings, or oil, divided
3   large potatoes, about 1 ½ pounds
1   medium yam or sweet potato, about 1 ½ pounds
    salt & pepper to taste
1   pound smoked turkey, or ham, cut into a ½ inch dice
1   medium onion (about 1 cup), cut into ½ inch pieces
1   tablespoon fresh chopped sage or 1 teaspoon dried sage
6   eggs

Preheat oven to 375 degrees. Prick potatoes and yam with a fork. On a small shallow pan, roast potatoes for 30 minutes. They should be firm and slightly underdone. Set aside until cool enough to handle. Peel yam. Cut potatoes and yam into a ½ inch dice (or grate them using a food processor shredder blade). Dicing looks better, but using the processor is faster.

Heat one of two large pans and add 2 tablespoons butter, bacon drippings, or oil. When bubbling subsides, add potatoes and yam. Sprinkle liberally with salt. Fry at medium high heat, stirring occasionally until evenly browned.

In the second large pan, brown smoked turkey in a remaining 1 tablespoon oil. Add diced onion. Stir to combine and cook until onion becomes translucent. Stir in sage.

Add smoked turkey mixture to the potatoes. Gently stir to combine. Keep pan on medium high heat and crack eggs over the top of the hash. Cover with a lid for one minute until eggs are soft-set. Spoon up servings of hash with one egg atop each portion. Garnish with sage.

Winter Citrus Salad with Pomegranate & Gingered Yogurt

Serves 6-8

Reducing the water content in the yogurt makes it thick and unbelievably creamy. Allow enough time to drain the yogurt overnight. To save time, purchase pre-drained Greek yogurt in specialty markets. A thickened yogurt recipe can be found in the "Other Stuff" section.

*Chinese five-spice powder and crystallized ginger are available in most supermarkets, some gourmet markets, and in Asian markets.

3   large oranges, all peel and pith cut away (pith is the bitter white stuff between the fruit and the peel)
1   grapefruit, peeled
4   clementines or small tangerines, peeled
1   pomegranate or ¼ cup dried sweetened cranberries
2   tablespoons honey
1   pinch Chinese five-spice powder*, or use a pinch each of black pepper and cardamom powder
1   pound plain whole milk yogurt
¼   cup minced crystallized ginger* (optional)
¼   teaspoon powdered ginger
¼   teaspoon ground cinnamon
2   tablespoons brown sugar, plus extra for garnish if desired

Drain yogurt in refrigerator overnight in sieve set over a medium bowl. Cut oranges into ½ inch rounds, then slice rounds into quarters. Separate grapefruit sections and cut each into ½ inch pieces. Remove any seeds. Cut clementines into ½ inch rounds, then slice in half. Combine oranges, grapefruit, and clementines in a large mixing bowl with all their juices.

Prepare pomegranate:

Cut pomegranate in half. Submerge in a deep bowl of water and break white pith away from seeds. Pith will float to the top and seeds will sink to the bottom. Add ¼-cup seeds to the orange mixture and reserve remaining seeds for another use, or add dried cranberries. Stir in honey and five-spice powder. Cover and refrigerate until ready to serve.

Stir drained yogurt with crystallized ginger (if using), ground ginger, cinnamon, and brown sugar. Cover and chill. (Fruit and yogurt can be made 1 day ahead). Spoon yogurt over fruit and serve.

For extra-special presentation, arrange fruit topped with yogurt in oven-proof casserole dish. Sprinkle brown sugar over top and broil in oven 3-4 minutes until sugar browns. Fruit will not be hot.

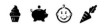

Breakfast Scones

Makes 20-22 scones

These scones are similar to the ones I made while working at Cucina Restaurant & Deli, in Salt Lake City, Utah. At the time, the kitchen was under the direction of talented chef-owner Marguerite Henderson. To give the scones more flavor and a little more rustic texture, this variation includes whole-wheat pastry flour and buttermilk in the glaze. Although they are sweeter than proper English scones, you will get nothing but compliments, even from friends from "across the pond." For ease of preparation, they cannot be beat.

For easy at-home scone "mix," combine the butter with the dry ingredients and keep refrigerated, or frozen, in a sealed container for up to several weeks. Anytime you wish to have hot, oven-fresh scones, simply add the half-n-half and your choice of flavorings and bake. This recipe is perfect when you want to give the kids a kitchen chore in the hot part of the day—without heating up the oven. They get their hands in the flour and rub in the butter. Then, you bake the next day in the cool of the morning. Your slumber-party breakfast will be a winner!

*Whole-wheat pastry flour is more finely ground than regular whole-wheat flour, making it ideal for tender pastry and baked goods. As a bonus, and in contrast to white flour, it also retains the texture and nutritional values of whole wheat. It is available in the bulk-food bins of most supermarkets and natural foods stores.

5 cups all-purpose unbleached flour
1 cup whole-wheat pastry flour*
1 ½ cups sugar
1 ½ tablespoons baking powder
1 teaspoon baking soda

1 teaspoon salt

¾ pound cold unsalted butter (3 sticks) cut in ½ inch pieces

2 ¼ cups half-and-half (use more if necessary)

Fruit flavorings (choose one):   1 pint raspberries

1 pint blueberries

1-2 cups sliced strawberries

1 pint blackberries

zest & juice of one orange + 1 cup pecans

2 mashed bananas +1 cup chocolate chips

1 cup raisins + 1 tablespoon cinnamon

1 cup sliced almonds + 1 teaspoon almond extract

1 cup poppy seeds + zest of one lemon

1 cup chopped apple + 1 tablespoon pie spice

1 cup pitted cherries

or make your own yummy combination

Glaze:

2   cups powdered sugar

¼   cup whole milk

2   tablespoons buttermilk

Mix first six ingredients in a large mixing bowl. With pastry cutter or processor cutting blade, cut butter into flour mixture until it is the size of small chunks. If using processor, pulse lightly. Dump mixture into a large mixing bowl. Using your fingers, rub butter into flour until the lumps are the size of peas and the butter is uniformly distributed. (Kids love this activity!) At this point, store the "mix" in a zip-loc bag or sealed container and refrigerate or freeze until ready to use.

To continue recipe, preheat oven to 375 degrees. In a large mixing bowl make a well in center of mix and pour in half-and-half and whatever fruit you choose. Mix gently to incorporate all liquid. Mixture will be lumpy. Do not over mix or scones will be tough! Scoop ½ cup mounds of batter onto parchment-lined baking sheet. Do not crowd baking sheet because scones will expand. Bake 25 minutes or until slightly golden. Cool slightly.

Whisk sugar, milk, and buttermilk together in a medium bowl and brush generously over still-warm scones to glaze. Serve warm or at room temperature. Can be made up to 8 hours in advance. Store in a sealed container in the refrigerator.

Tammy's Granola

Makes 12 cups

I eat this every morning with milk and a cup of herb tea. It is powerful food.

*Feel free to experiment with your favorite additions. Try amaranth, golden flax seeds, or any other seed. Alternative grains are available in health food stores. Particularly good are millet, rolled barley, or quinoa. As long as whole grains are rolled or chopped fine, they can be added. Try natural maple syrup in place of some of the honey. Sprinkle cinnamon or other spices on the oats before baking. Let your imagination go wild.

In big microwave-safe mixing bowl mix together:

2 cups brown sugar

1 cup honey

⅓ cup water

Microwave sugar mixture on high for five minutes. It will become liquid caramel. Watch carefully, it will bubble up. Remove from microwave and add:

3 teaspoons vanilla

1 teaspoon salt

In an extremely large mixing bowl, combine together:

10 cups rolled oats or seven-grain mix

6 cups nuts & seeds (almonds, walnuts, sunflower seeds, pumpkin seeds, sesame seeds, flax seeds, millet, quinoa, bran flakes, wheat germ, etc.*)

4 cups shredded coconut (unsweetened)

Pour hot caramel over oat mixture and stir to coat. Spread granola evenly in a single layer in four un-greased cookie sheets.

Bake sheets at 275° in upper and lower oven racks for 45 minutes, and up to one hour, rotating pans halfway through cooking to produce even browning. When cooled, scrape granola into a large bowl with metal spatula. Add dried fruit if desired: raisins, currants, sultanas, apricot, prune, fig, date, mango, pineapple, banana, pear, apple, cherry, etc.

Store in airtight container in the refrigerator to keep the nuts and seeds fresh.

⚡ ⏰ ☺

Mango Lassi (Indian Mango-Yogurt Drink)

Serves 2

Lassi is a very popular drink both in India and Pakistan. It is available not only from roadside cafés but is also a great favorite in good restaurants and hotels. There is no substitute for this drink, especially on a hot day. It is ideal served with hot dishes as it cools the palette and helps digest spicy food. Other fresh fruit purées can be substituted for mango, including passion-fruit, guava, and berries of all kinds. Try it for breakfast as a jump-start alternative to coffee.

1 cup natural (plain) lowfat or whole milk yogurt
2 tablespoons sugar, or to taste
6 ice cubes
¼ cup ice water
3 tablespoons puréed mango or 1 fresh medium mango, peeled, pitted, and cut into chunks
1 tablespoon crushed pistachio nuts

If using fresh mango chunks, puree fruit in a blender until smooth. Add to mango puree: sugar, ice cubes, and ice water and blend until smooth. Pour into chilled serving glasses and garnish with crushed pistachio nuts. Serve cold.

Seasonal Salads

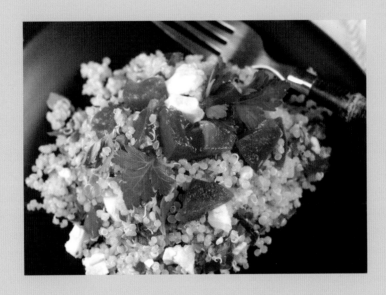

Lemon Couscous Salad with Spinach, Feta, & Mint

page 171

Springtime Salads

Green Things Salad

Serves 6-8

For this mixed salad, look for fresh seasonal vegetables. Get adventurous and try less common items including shredded Brussels sprouts, okra, chopped broccoli stems, edename (soybeans), mâche (small, clover-shaped sprouted greens), fava beans, or chopped kohlrabi. For those of you new to kohlrabi, it looks like something from a swampy planet outside our solar system—but it is delicious. Toss with elegant avocado dressing for a healthful send-up to green vegetables.

Ingredients

8 cups mixed salad greens

3 green onions, minced

1-2 cups chopped green vegetables (broccoli florets, cucumbers, zucchini, spinach, green beans, sprouts, celery, etc.)

Dressing
1 large ripe avocado
grated peel and juice of 1 lime
1 clove garlic, crushed
1 teaspoon honey
salt and pepper
4 tablespoons of milk (or more)
chopped parsley

Method

Wash greens and spin dry. Use a salad spinner, or, as my friend Heather taught me, throw wet greens in an old pillow case and twirl the bag around your head until dry. This method tends to fling water, so it is suggested to do this outside, preferably where the neighbors won't see you. Toss greens with green onions and chopped vegetables. Can be prepared 2-3 hours ahead. Cover and refrigerate.

For dressing:

Halve avocado, remove pit, and scoop flesh out into blender or food processor. Add grated lime peel, lime juice, garlic, honey, salt, pepper, and 2 tablespoons of milk. Blend until smooth. Thin with remaining milk if necessary. Arrange salad on individual serving plates. Top with a big dollop of avocado dressing and sprinkle with parsley.

Lemon Couscous Salad with Spinach, Feta, & Mint

Serves 6

This is perfect to make a day ahead because the flavors improve as it sits overnight.

3⅓ cups water
2¼ cups couscous (about 15 ounces)
1 teaspoon salt
4 tablespoons fresh lemon juice
½ cup extra virgin olive oil
3 cups spinach, cleaned, dried, and chopped fine
3 large green onions (scallions), chopped fine
3 tablespoons fresh mint, chopped fine
2 ounces crumbled feta cheese
½ cucumber, peeled, seeded and chopped fine
2 tablespoons sun-dried tomatoes packed in oil, drained, and chopped fine

Bring water to a boil in a saucepan and stir in couscous and salt. Remove pan from heat and let couscous stand, covered, 5 minutes. Fluff couscous with a fork and transfer to a bowl. Stir in lemon juice, oil, and salt and pepper to taste and cool completely.

Stir in spinach, green onions, mint, feta, cucumber and sun-dried tomatoes and chill salad, covered at least 2 hours, or overnight.

Savory Summer Cole Slaw

Serves 10

The colors of this coleslaw are beautiful and appetizing. Stir well after refrigerating to redistribute dressing. You can double or triple this recipe for a large crowd.

Substitutions are permissible in almost all salad recipes. Bottled lemon juice can be used in place of fresh lemon juice. Yellow mustard works in place of Dijon. Poppy seeds or anise seeds can stand in for celery seeds. Does the final product taste the same? Not exactly—but who cares as long as it remains delicious. Besides, cooking without fuss is a pleasure.

½ large head green cabbage
½ head small purple cabbage
2 large carrots, peeled
4 large green onions (scallions), root-end trimmed—which means cut off the hairy part
1 small green bell pepper, or half of a large pepper
6-8 large red radishes
½ sweet purple onion

Dressing

1½ cup mayonnaise
1 clove garlic minced
juice of 1 large lemon (about 1 ½ tablespoons or to taste)
1 tablespoon Dijon mustard
2 tablespoons celery seed
¼ cup sugar
salt and pepper to taste

Using processor, shred cabbages, carrots, scallions, bell pepper, radishes, and purple onion. Toss together in a very large bowl.

In a medium bowl, whisk together dressing ingredients. Season dressing with salt and pepper to taste. Add more sugar if necessary. It should taste savory, salty, sweet, and lemony.

Pour dressing over coleslaw and stir well. Refrigerate for several hours before serving. This coleslaw is excellent served the next day after the flavors have melded together.

Tabouli

Serves six

This salad boasts bright, fresh flavors that are addictive and healthy. The individual elements of this recipe can be prepped ahead of time and combined just before serving. Garbanzo beans are an unusual addition, adding protein and fiber to round out this nutritionally jam-packed dish.

*Tabouli is an ancient food common to the Middle East and Mediterranean countries. The primary component of Tabouli is bulgar wheat. Despite its unappetizing name, bulgar is versatile and delicious because it is essentially cracked whole-wheat—the kind that can be made into cereal. In this recipe, the cooked bulgar absorbs the lemon, garlic, and olive oil flavors and provides a savory-nutty base for the vegetables. Think of it as a close cousin to rice pilaf or couscous. Look for bulgar in the grains, rice, and beans section of your supermarket, or in the bulk food bins of health food stores. Bulgar is often sold as a boxed Tabouli mix with flavorings (mostly salt) already added. Use pre-packaged Tabouli only if you cannot find plain bulgar, and taste first before adding any extra salt.

1 cup dry bulgar or whole wheat couscous
1½ cup boiling water
1 teaspoon salt
¼ cup fresh lemon juice
¼ cup olive oil
2 cloves garlic, minced
pepper to taste
2 tomatoes, chopped
½ cup garbanzo beans, drained and rinsed
½ cup bell pepper, chopped
1 small cucumber, seeded and diced
¼ cup fresh parsley, washed and chopped
4 scallions, chopped

In a small pot, pour boiling water over bulgar. Cover and let stand for 30 minutes.

Combine salt, lemon juice, olive oil, garlic, and pepper. Mix well. Stir vinaigrette into cooked bulgar. Refrigerate until cold. Can be made one day in advance.

Stir in remaining ingredients right before serving. If needed, adjust seasoning with more salt and pepper, and serve.

Fall Salads

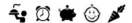

Apple Waldorf Salad

Serves 6

Sometimes I just need a Waldorf! I prefer full-fat, inexpensive off-brand mayonnaise made with canola oil. Avoid lowfat or fat free mayo because they taste bad and make the dressing watery. Better to have a little fat and enjoy it, than to have a pile of inferior salad.

3 medium tart apples, traditionally Granny Smith
3 stalks celery
¼ cup dried cranberries or seedless grapes, halved
½ cup walnuts
1 head butter lettuce

Dressing
½ cup mayonnaise
juice of ½ lemon, plus extra to prevent apples from browning (about 2 teaspoons)
1 teaspoon sugar
freshly ground pepper

Preheat oven to 375 degrees and toast walnuts in a shallow pan for 10 minutes until fragrant. Allow nuts to cool. Coarsely chop walnuts.

Wash and core apples, leaving the peel on. Chop them into 1 inch pieces. Place them in a large mixing bowl. Sprinkle lemon juice over apples to keep from browning. Dice celery into ½ inch pieces and add to apples. Add cranberries and walnuts to apple mixture. Toss to combine. Wash and spin dry lettuce (see "Green Things Salad" recipe above for low-tech salad-spinning solutions), keeping whole leaves intact.

In a medium mixing bowl, whisk dressing ingredients to combine. Pour dressing over apple mixture. Mix gently. Refrigerate until ready to serve.

Place a whole lettuce leaf on each place. Spoon apple salad into center of leaf. Serve.

Roasted Beet Salad with Pear, Arugula, & Bleu Cheese

Serves 6

Oven roasting beets concentrates their flavors and yields sweet, silky flesh with a transcendent burst of flavor. You can buy fancy heirloom varieties with unusual colors and sizes, but plain old red beets are just as good. When you must, substitute canned beets, but do not hesitate to try roasting fresh beets because it could not be easier.

*Arugula leaves are either rounded like spinach or shaped like an oak-leaf. When harvested young, they have a nice peppery taste similar to a radish. Arugula is sweeter, milder, and more tender during cooler spring and fall months than during hot months. Spinach makes a nice stand-in for arugula.

3 pounds beets
8 cups arugula* or spinach, washed and spun dry (see "Green Things Salad" for spin tips)
3 pears
1 cup walnuts
½ small red onion, sliced into thin rings
½ cup bleu cheese or goat cheese, crumbled

Dressing

¼ cup sherry vinegar
1 tablespoon lemon juice

¼ cup orange juice
1 tablespoon water
½ cup extra virgin olive oil
salt and pepper

Preheat oven to 375 degrees. Rinse beets of any noticeable dirt. Trim off green tops if attached. On a parchment-lined baking sheet, roast beets with the skin on for about 45 minutes to an hour. Place walnuts on a separate pie plate and roast in same oven with beets for about 10 minutes until browning and fragrant. Remove walnuts. Check beets after 45 minutes by inserting fork or thin knife-blade into thickest part. When blade comes out easily, beets are done. Cool beets and walnuts.

Cut pears in half length-wise (north to south). Using a spoon or melon baller, remove inner core with seeds. Using paring knife, remove stem and blossom ends. Place pear cut-side down and cut lengthwise into thin slices. Arrange slices in concentric circles on a serving platter or on individual plates. Arrange several onion rings over pear, extending out to the edges of the fruit.

Peel cooled beets. Slice big beets into large rounds, and slice small beets into quarters. Arrange beet slices in the middle so the pear is showing.

In a small mixing bowl whisk vinegar, lemon juice, orange juice, and water to combine. Drizzle in olive oil, whisking vigorously until oil in emulsified. Correct seasoning with salt and pepper. The dressing should have a nice bright balance of salty, sweet, and tangy.

Place arugula in a large bowl and toss with enough dressing to lightly coat greens. Mound greens in the center on top of beets. Sprinkle with toasted walnuts and crumbled bleu cheese. Drizzle salad with a little extra dressing. Serve.

Curried Chicken-Apricot-Walnut Salad in Lettuce Cups

Yield: about 20 appetizers and 2 cups salad

This recipe gives you plenty of extra salad. Try it stuffed in croissants or rolls for a terrific lunch. Cut recipe in half if you don't want leftover salad.

To serve as a buffet salad, line a large platter with lettuce and mound salad in the center. Garnish with oranges and cilantro for a beautiful presentation.

*Belgium endive is actually grown in the dark. It originated as the accidental offshoot of the chicory root but is now actively cultivated for its crunchy leaves, silky texture, and pleasantly bitter taste. The tightly closed capsule-shaped heads can be separated into individual spears, just the right size for filling.

1 lb boneless, skinless cooked chicken breasts, cut into ½ inch dice (bite-sized pieces)
2 stalks celery, finely minced
¼ cup toasted walnuts, chopped
½ cup dried apricots, finely chopped

Dressing
1 cup mayonnaise
2 tablespoons curry powder
½ teaspoon cinnamon
½ teaspoon ground cumin
⅓ cup brown sugar
1 teaspoon salt
½ teaspoon white pepper
2-3 large heads Belgium endive* (or use a combination of radicchio, romaine hearts, Boston lettuce hearts or other lettuce varieties).

In a large bowl, combine chicken with celery, walnuts, and apricots. In a separate bowl, whisk dressing ingredients until well blended. Pour dressing over chicken mixture and stir to combine. Refrigerate salad until ready to serve—at least one hour and up to one day.

Prepare lettuce cups by carefully separating heads and washing and drying individual lettuce cups. Spoon heaping tablespoons of salad into each cup. Serve.

Parisian Salad with Cured Salmon, Pink Grapefruit, & Fennel

Serves 4-6 as a side dish

My husband and I were treated to this classic winter salad by wonderful friends from Paris. The acid in the grapefruit is the perfect foil for the richness of the salmon. If you don't like fish, substitute shaved proscuitto or other good-quality cured ham. Feel free to use blood oranges (because they are tart) as an excellent alternative to grapefruit.

* Fennel looks a bit like celery with a white bulb at the bottom and fronds at the top. When raw, it has a pleasant licorice anise taste. When cooked, it mellows and become sweet. Fennel is sometimes labeled "anise" and is found in most produce sections.

1 large head butter (Boston) lettuce
¼ sweet red onion
1-2 ripe pink grapefruit
1 lb good-quality cured salmon, sliced thin
½ fresh fennel bulb* (stalk and fronds trimmed), or substitute with Belgium endive
1 lemon, juiced
1 tablespoon Dijon mustard
2 tablespoon water
½ cup olive oil
salt & pepper

Wash and dry lettuce. Peel grapefruit. Working over a bowl to catch juices, divide grapefruit sections, removing membranes between each section. Reserve grapefruit sections. Squeeze remaining grapefruit pulp and membranes to release juices. Set aside juices. Slice onion into narrow strips. Slice fennel into narrow strips—a mandoline slicer or standing slicer works well to produce very thin slices of onion and fennel.

Vinaigrette

In small bowl, whisk lemon juice, mustard, and water. Add any reserved juices from grapefruit segments. Correct seasoning with salt and fresh ground pepper. Continue whisking and slowly add oil in small stream. Dressing is complete when all oil is added and dressing is emulsified.

Toss lettuce with enough vinaigrette to coat. Divide the lettuce between plates. Arrange salmon, onion, fennel, and grapefruit sections atop lettuce on each plate. Drizzle more vinaigrette over composed salad. Pass extra dressing separately.

Variation:
Garnish top of salad with sprigs of dill or a small bunch of washed machê (a small green sprout resembling clover). Capers can also be strewn about the salad for garnish. In addition, roasted almonds, walnuts, and pecans go well with this dish.

Main Courses

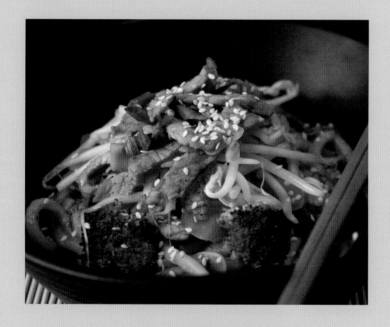

Beef & Broccoli with Black Bean & Garlic Sauce
page 182

Stir Fry 3 Ways

Because stir-fry is such an easy way to enjoy vegetables, I have included three variations. As you become familiar with the flavor profiles of each sauce, try plugging in whatever meat and vegetable components light you up. For instance, peppers and lamb are great in the chili-garlic sauce. Tofu, mushrooms, and leeks work well in the ginger sauce. Red snapper and Napa cabbage taste delicious in the black bean and garlic sauce. Discover your own favorite combinations. Serve stir-fry with brown rice, basmati rice, or jasmine rice.

Beef & Broccoli with Black Bean & Garlic Sauce

Serves 2-4

* Black Bean and Garlic Sauce is a dark, rich, and salty fermented bean sauce. Try it mixed into buttered green beans for a savory side dish. You can find this sauce in the Asian aisle of most supermarkets.

Marinade
2 teaspoons soy sauce
1 tablespoon fresh ginger, minced fine, or 1 teaspoon dried ground ginger
2 teaspoons dry sherry or rice wine
1 tablespoon cornstarch

Stir Fry Ingredients
3 tablespoons peanut oil
½ pound beef, thinly sliced—use any cut of beef because the marinade will tenderize meat
2 pounds broccoli, washed, florets separated from stalks and cut into 1-inch pieces
½ green pepper, cut into pieces
½ yellow onion, cut into pieces
1 cup fresh bean sprouts
2 tablespoons black bean and garlic sauce*
1 tablespoon oyster sauce (available in most markets)

In a small bowl, combine beef with marinade ingredients. Allow meat mixture to rest at room temperature at least 10 minutes and up to ½ hour.

Heat oil in wok. Add beef, and chow (stir) until seared, but not cooked all the way through. Remove meat to a bowl and set aside. Without wiping out wok, add broccoli florets, green pepper, onion, and Black Bean and Garlic Sauce, and stir-fry for 2 minutes. Add 1 cup water and cover with lid. Simmer covered one minute, or until broccoli is bright green and crisp-tender. Return beef to wok. Add bean sprouts. Stir until beef is cooked to desired doneness, mixture is shiny, and sauce is slightly thickened.

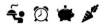

Chinese Greens with Light Ginger Sauce

Serves 2-4

Chinese cuisine utilizes a wide spectrum of greens and this recipe features tender pea shoots. Harvested when they are only a few inches tall, they are small round leaves with thin stems. Look for bags of fresh greens in your Asian market. As a substitute, use baby bok choy, Napa cabbage, or spinach.

Sauce
2 tablespoons peanut oil
1 garlic clove, minced
1 tablespoon fresh ginger, minced or 1 teaspoon ground dried ginger
1 tablespoon oyster sauce (available in most markets)
½ teaspoon sugar
1 tablespoon cornstarch
¼ cup water
1 pound Chinese greens, washed and chopped
*Optional—toasted sesame oil

Heat oil in wok. Add garlic and ginger. Stir for 30 seconds, do not brown. Add greens, oyster sauce, and sugar. Stir-fry until greens turn bright green and begin to wilt. Add spoonfuls of water if dry.

In small bowl mix 2 teaspoons cornstarch in a little water to dissolve. Pour cornstarch mixture over greens and stir until sauce becomes shiny and coats greens. Add a few drops of sesame oil if desired.

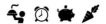

Chili-Garlic Shrimp with Green Beans, Carrots, & Mushrooms

Serves 2-4

Because it only takes minutes to stir-fry, prep all ingredients before you start cooking. Cut ingredients into similar shapes and sizes for uniformity of cooking time and ease of eating. Each component of stir-fry should be cooked just until crisp-tender. To prevent overcooking the fish, shrimp, or meat, precook and then combine the cooked ingredients at the end because the vegetables require more time over heat than the proteins.

*To reconstitute dried mushrooms, soak them in a bowl of boiling water. Dried mushrooms float so you may need to set a smaller dish directly on top as a weight to keep them submerged. Some mushrooms are tougher than others and may require up to 30 minutes soaking time to soften woody stems. Discard stems if they remain tough. When draining mushrooms, reserve the flavorful soaking liquid for use in cooking. Because mushrooms can render dirt into the soaking liquid, allow a minute for the grit to settle at the bottom of the bowl. Then, pour liquid out, being careful to leave sediment undisturbed at the bottom.

*Ginger can be chopped like any firm vegetable—no need to peel it unless it has a particularly ugly blemish on the skin. The peel will not be noticeable in the final product. Fresh ginger keeps well wrapped in plastic in the refrigerator for a week or two.

*The heat of fresh chilies comes from the chemical capsicum, which is concentrated primarily in the white membranes and seeds inside the chili. To control the heat, remove the desired amount of seeds and ribs with a sharp paring knife. You may want to wear gloves for this task. Bird's eye chilies are red with some green coloration and are found in most Asian markets. Jalapeños or serranos make good substitutes.

*Hoisin sauce is a dark sweet-tangy sauce found in the Asian section of most supermarkets. Try it brushed on baked chicken with a little garlic.

*Sambal is an Indonesian chili sauce made from hot chilies, garlic, and vinegar. Each region, and for that matter each Indonesian grandmother, has their own special formula for this multi-purpose sauce. Sambal can be found in the Asian section of most supermarkets.

Stir Fry Ingredients
3 tablespoons peanut oil
1 pound raw shrimp, peeled (see instructions below)

1 carrot, cut into 2 inch long julienne strips (very thin, like matchsticks)
½ pound green beans, washed and stemmed, cut into 2 inch lengths
5 large fresh shitake mushrooms, cut into thin strips (or use reconstituted dried mushrooms)*

Sauce
2 cloves garlic, minced
1 teaspoon fresh ginger*, minced, or ½ teaspoon dried ground ginger
2 Thai bird's eye chilies*, or other hot chili, stemmed, seeded and diced fine
2 teaspoons hoisin sauce*
½ teaspoon sambal (Indonesian chili sauce)*
pinch of sugar (a pinch is generally about ⅛ teaspoon)
¼ cup water
1 tablespoon cornstarch
¼ cup water

To thaw frozen shrimp, place in a colander in sink and periodically run cold water over it until soft. To peel thawed shrimp, first remove legs and main shell, and then carefully pull off tail, leaving tail meat intact.

Heat oil in wok. Add shrimp and stir until it turns pink and is almost cooked through (as it cooks, raw shrimp loses its gray transparency and becomes opaque). Remove shrimp to a bowl. Add carrots, green beans, and shitake mushrooms. Stir 1 minute. Add all remaining ingredients except cornstarch and shrimp. Stir for 2 minutes, and add shrimp. Add ¼ cup water if dry.

Mix cornstarch with ¼ cup water and stir into shrimp mixture. Cook until sauce is shiny and thickened, about 1 minute. Serve with rice or noodles.

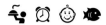

Teriyaki-Caramel Glazed Salmon

Makes 2 cups teriyaki sauce; serves 4 entrees

I developed this recipe while working at an upscale restaurant and deli. It immediately became a customer favorite and standard menu item at the restaurant. Try this sauce brushed over grilled tofu squares for a great vegetarian entrée.

2 cups brown sugar
½ cup soy sauce
1 teaspoon ginger, ground
2 teaspoons minced garlic

2-3 pounds salmon fillets
blonde or black sesame seeds for garnish

Preheat oven to 375 degrees. In a deep heavy pot, combine brown sugar, soy sauce, ginger, and garlic. Heat to a boil while stirring. Allow mixture to bubble and boil until slightly thickened and shiny (about 3-5 minutes). Set aside. If mixture becomes too thick just thin with a little water.

On a parchment-lined baking sheet arrange salmon fillets. Bake until almost cooked through (about 6 minutes). Remove salmon from oven and brush teriyaki caramel generously over fish. Return to oven and finish cooking 1-2 minutes more. Do not overcook fish. Drizzle with more teriyaki sauce. Sprinkle with sesame seeds to garnish. Any extra sauce can be served alongside fish. Serve with rice and vegetables.

Sea Scallops Primavera

Serves four

This recipe is both light and flavorful. Don't be put off by the large list of ingredients—it comes together quickly.

*Leeks are members of the onion family with a lovely savory-rich quality when cooked. Their white inch-wide stalks and green tops collect a lot of dirt, so separate and wash each stalk thoroughly. Use the white part and 1-2 inches into the green part. Leeks are at their peak in the spring, but are available year-round in the produce section of the grocery store.

*Shallots are related to garlic and have a potent flavor similar to a cross between onion and garlic. Like onions and ogres, shallots have layers and a papery outer skin. Raw minced shallot is typically used in vinaigrette salad dressings. Shallots bring depth and complexity to a myriad of cooked dishes ranging from sauces, soups, pastas, and this seafood entrée.

1 pound sea scallops
1 teaspoon olive oil
salt and pepper to taste
1 medium leek*, cleaned and minced fine
2 small shallots*, peeled and minced fine
1 clove garlic, peeled and minced fine
1 cup parsley, washed and minced fine
juice of ½ lemon
1 tablespoon soy sauce
1 cube fish bouillon, dissolved in 1 cup hot water

¼ sweet red bell pepper, chopped
¼ green bell pepper, chopped
½ large carrot, chopped
6 large mushrooms, chopped
1 stalk celery, chopped

½ teaspoon fresh ginger, minced (or ¼ teaspoon ground dried ginger)
1 tablespoon fresh dill, chopped (or ½ tablespoon dried)
2 tablespoons fresh cilantro, chopped

Heat large fry pan with olive oil. Sauté scallops until just opaque, approximately two minutes per side. Season scallops with salt and pepper to taste. Remove scallops to a plate and cover with foil to keep warm.

In same skillet, sauté chopped leek, shallot, garlic, and parsley, adding more oil if necessary. Sauté for only 2-3 minutes. Add lemon juice, soy sauce, and fish bouillon cube dissolved in the hot water. Bring to a simmer.

Add peppers, carrot, mushrooms, and celery to skillet. Cook vegetables just until crisp-tender and colors are bright. Add minced ginger. Return scallops to the skillet with any juices. When scallops are hot, add chopped dill and cilantro. Serve immediately with rice.

Chicken

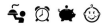

Easy Apricot Chicken

Contributed by Michelle Sundwall – Serves about 6

What could be easier than dumping chicken in a crock pot with three other ingredients? The best part is you can leave it unattended all day and come home to tender, savory chicken. Soprano Michelle Sundwall shared this recipe on my radio show, Get Real Food, *with Gourmet Tres, and it has been a favorite ever since. With its savory-sweet flavor profile, this chicken goes well with rice pilaf as an accompaniment.*

2 fryer chickens cut up (about 3 pounds) or 2 ½ pounds boneless chicken breast tenders
1 (8 ounce) bottle Russian or French Salad Dressing
1 cup apricot jam
1 package dry onion soup mix

Crock Pot Method:
In a crock-pot mix salad dressing, jam, and soup mix. Add chicken and stir to combine. Simmer on low until tender.

Oven Method:

Preheat oven to 350 degrees. In a large casserole dish, combine salad dressing, jam, and onion soup mix. Add chicken and stir to coat chicken. Bake uncovered for about an hour until chicken is cooked through.

*Serving Suggestion: Serve with a rice pilaf made from rice cooked in chicken broth with a handful of raisins, chopped green onions, and sliced almonds.

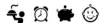

Honey-Lime-Ginger Chicken

Serve 2-4 entrees

Serve this with a green salad, sliced pineapple, and steamed quinoa for an easy, healthy meal.

Tenderized chicken cooks uniformly and has an improved texture. To tenderize chicken breasts, place each piece between two pieces of plastic wrap, or in a re-closeable bag. Using a meat-tenderizing mallet or the flat end of a heavy can, pound thickest parts of chicken until the whole piece is of uniform thickness.

The outer peel of lemons, limes, oranges, and grapefruit is called the "zest" because it contains the fragrant oils and pronounced citrus flavors of the fruit. Use a citrus zester or a grater to remove only the outer colored part of the peel, avoiding the bitter white pith inside the peel.

Ingredients
2 teaspoons butter, divided
2 teaspoons olive oil
1 pound boneless, skinless chicken breast (about 2 breast halves), tenderized*

¼ cup liquid (chicken stock, water, fruit juice, herb tea, white wine, etc.)
1 heaping tablespoon honey
1 teaspoon ginger, minced
2 large garlic cloves, minced
juice and zest* of half a lime (or more)
1 teaspoon Dijon mustard
1 teaspoon soy sauce

Preheat oven to 350 degrees.

Heat medium, (oven-safe) sauté pan on medium high. Sprinkle chicken breasts with salt. Add 1 teaspoon butter and oil and when oil is hot, brown chicken in pan, turning once after 2 minutes.

Add all other ingredients to pan, stirring liquids with a whisk. Pan will steam and bubble vigorously. Take pan off heat and cover loosely with foil.

Bake in oven until chicken is cooked through, approximately 7-10 more minutes. Carefully take pan out of oven and transfer chicken to a plate (pan handle is HOT). Do not clean pan. Return same pan with cooking juices to the stove. Reduce sauce by boiling down liquids until thickened and shiny, about 2 minutes, whisking constantly. Remove sauce from stove and whisk in remaining 1 teaspoon butter (to give sauce body, flavor, and shine). Serve chicken, spooning sauce over top. Garnish with lime wedge and cilantro sprig if desired.

Penne with Lemon Chicken, Artichokes, & Olives

Serves 4

This easy one-pot dish turns leftover rotisserie chicken or canned chicken into a real treat. Use either oil-marinated artichoke hearts or the kind in brine. If using the kind in oil, reserve a few tablespoons of the marinade and add it to the pasta for extra flavor. Serve with a green salad.

1 pound penne (or other short pasta)
¼ cup olive oil
1 garlic clove, minced fine
1 teaspoon lemon pepper
½ cup pitted kalamata olives (dark brown Greek olives)
2 (6 ounce) jars artichoke hearts, oil marinade reserved, brine drained
2 cups coarsely chopped cooked chicken—or, omit chicken for a vegetarian entree
½ cup grated Parmesan or Asiago cheese

In a large pot, heat 8 cups of water to a rolling boil. Salt water with 2 teaspoons salt and add penne, stirring occasionally. Drain pasta when penne is quite al dente (a little undercooked). Return pasta to hot pot and add all other ingredients, sprinkling the lemon pepper evenly over pasta. Toss gently over medium heat to heat through, and serve.

Portobello Mushrooms
with Barley Risotto & Basil-Tomato Salsa

Makes 6 servings

Who would believe this elegant entrée is also vegetarian? Similar in texture to Italian risotto made with rice, this variation instead features barley. This dish easily converts for vegan diets by substituting oil for the butter and using soy cheese.

*Pearl barley is found in the dried bean and grain aisle of the supermarket.

Barley Risotto
6 ½ cups low-salt vegetable or chicken broth
4 tablespoons unsalted butter
1 medium onion, finely chopped
2 medium garlic cloves, minced
2 cups pearl barley* (about 13 ounces), rinsed, drained

Portobello Mushrooms
6 (3 inch diameter) Portobello mushrooms, wiped free of dirt, stems removed
½ cup freshly grated parmesan cheese (about 1 ½ ounces)
1 tablespoon chopped fresh chives
1 tablespoon chopped fresh Italian parsley

Basil-tomato Salsa
4 large Roma tomatoes (about 1 ½ pounds), coarsely chopped
1 tablespoon extra-virgin olive oil
1 large clove garlic, minced
6 large basil leaves, coarsely chopped

Melt 2 tablespoons butter in heavy large saucepan over medium heat. Add onion and garlic; sauté until tender, about 6 minutes. Add barley; stir until coated with butter, about 1 minute. Add ½ cup broth; simmer, stirring often, until broth is absorbed, about 3 minutes. Add remaining broth in several additions, allowing most of the broth to be absorbed before adding more, stirring frequently until barley is tender but still firm and barley risotto is creamy, about 45 minutes total.

Meanwhile, preheat oven to 375 degrees. Arrange mushroom caps gills-down on a parchment-lined baking sheet. Brush mushroom tops with olive oil. Roast for 15-20 minutes until color darkens and mushrooms are firm-tender. Season to taste with salt and pepper.

Combine chopped tomatoes, olive oil, garlic, and basil in a small bowl. Season to taste with salt and pepper. Set aside at room temperature.

Add to risotto parmesan cheese, herbs, and remaining 2 tablespoons butter. Stir to combine. Season to taste with salt and pepper.

On six plates, spoon some tomato-basil salsa. Top with a mushroom, gills-side up. Spoon a generous portion of risotto over the mushroom. Garnish with extra parmesan cheese and additional salsa.

Skewered Zucchini-wrapped Fresh Mozzarella Balls with Bread Crumbs

Serves 6

This dish takes the yummy-ness of fried cheese to a whole new level. Personally, I think everything tastes better when you put it on a stick. If using bamboo skewers, soak them in water for at least 30 minutes prior to cooking so they don't smoke and burn.

*Look for bocconcini or large fresh mozzarella balls in Mediterranean markets and the cheese section of better grocery stores. Typically, they are stored in a milky water bath, which is drained before using. Inspect the expiration date. It should be fresh.

18 small fresh mozzarella balls (bocconcini)—or cut a full-size fresh mozzarella into eight wedges, drained
4 medium zucchini, about 1 inch wide
12 (1 inch) cherry or grape tomatoes
3 cups fresh bread crumbs (grind up day-old bread in processor)

½ cup butter
olive oil for brushing
salt and pepper
6 long metal or bamboo skewers

Preheat oven to 375 degrees. Using the ⅟₁₆ inch slicing blade of a mandoline (standing slicer), or a chef's knife, or with a vegetable peeler, cut long strips of unpeeled zucchini. You will need 18 strips total. In a large pot of salted, simmering water, blanche zucchini strips for 15 seconds until they are bright green and pliable. Remove quickly and plunge zucchini into a bowl of ice water to arrest cooking. Drain well.

On a work surface pat dry one zucchini strip with paper towels. Place a mozzarella ball, or wedge, on one end and roll up in zucchini. Thread skewer through the center of bundle to secure. Slide a cherry tomato next to the zucchini and mozzarella ball. Repeat with another mozzarella ball and add to skewer followed by another cherry tomato. Finish with a final zucchini-wrapped mozzarella. There should be 3 cheese bundles on each skewer. Continue with remaining 5 skewers. Place skewers in a large oiled casserole dish and brush them with olive oil. Season with salt and pepper.

In a large sauté pan, melt butter over medium heat. When foam subsides, add breadcrumbs and stir until butter is thoroughly mixed in and crumbs are golden brown.

Roast skewers in preheated oven 5 minutes until cheese begins to soften. Cover skewers with breadcrumbs and bake for another 5 minutes until crumbs are toasted and cheese is melted. Serve immediately directly from casserole dish. Accompany with a green salad for a tasty meal.

Chard & Feta Pie

Serves 8 as a side dish

Like the Greek finger food spanikopita, this pie has an herbed cheese filling surrounded by flaky phyllo dough. Fresh dill, greens, and feta cheese combine inside the pastry for a contemporary twist. Phyllo is remarkably thin and must be kept covered to prevent drying out. Cutting slits into the top phyllo layer allows steam to escape during baking so the crust will be crisp. To serve a larger crowd, double the recipe and bake the pies side by side in the oven. Serve with vegetable soup and crusty bread

Swiss Chard is a highly nutritious leafy plant, similar to collard greens. Although it looks like lettuce, it is a member of the cruciferous family, and is more closely related to cabbage and broccoli than it is to anything you might find in a salad. It cooks quickly and the tender, sweet leaves can be used interchangeably with spinach in soups and many other preparations. Chard leaves are usually green, but the veins and stems may range in color from white, to purple, to orange.

2 quarts water
12 cups torn Swiss chard* (about ¾ pound), washed
8 cups torn spinach (about ½ pound), washed
1 tablespoon olive oil
2 cups chopped Vidalia or other sweet onion
2 garlic cloves, minced
¼ cup chopped fresh dill
¼ cup chopped fresh flat-leaf parsley
¾ cup (3 ounces) crumbled feta cheese
2 large eggs, lightly beaten
2 large egg whites, lightly beaten
½ teaspoon freshly ground black pepper
¼ teaspoon salt

10 sheets frozen phyllo dough, thawed
Cooking Spray

Bring 2 quarts water to a boil in a large pot. Add the chard and cook 2 minutes or until tender. Add spinach, stirring until wilted, another 30 seconds. Drain well. Place chard and spinach on several layers of paper towels, squeezing until barely moist.

Preheat oven to 375 degrees. Heat oil in a large nonstick skillet over medium-high heat. Add onion; sauté 5 minutes or until tender. Add garlic; sauté 1 minute. Add chard mixture, dill, and parsley, stirring well to combine. Cook greens 1 minute until thoroughly heated. Remove from heat. Combine chard mixture, cheese, eggs, and egg whites, mixing well to combine. Stir in pepper and salt.

Place 1 phyllo sheet on a large cutting board or work surface. Cover remaining dough with plastic wrap to prevent drying. Lightly coat phyllo sheet with cooking spray. Coat a 9 inch pie plate with cooking spray and arrange phyllo sheet, oiled side up, in pie plate, allowing edges to hang over rim. Spray another sheet of phyllo and place directly on top of first sheet, in an offset pattern so corners do not align. Repeat the procedure with 5 more phyllo sheets, for a total of 7 sheets, alternating corners in a crisscross design. Spoon the spinach mixture over phyllo. Lightly coat each of the remaining 3 phyllo sheets with cooking spray, and place sheets over spinach mixture in a crisscross design. Using your hands, roll excess overhanging phyllo into the dish to create a crimped, sealed edge; press lightly to hold. Cut 4 (2 inch) slits in top of pie; cover with foil. Bake at 375 for 10 minutes. Uncover and bake an additional 30 minutes or until crust is crisp and golden. Cut pie into 8 wedges.

Lentils with Onion-Tomato Marmalade

Serves 4-6 as a side dish

My family has enjoyed this Indian dish countless times. It is meatless, but so full of protein and complex flavor you can serve it as a main course. Double the recipe to yield enough for entrée portions. Try adding diced carrot, celery, peas, or diced potato for variations. To give it a French twist, omit the turmeric and replace it with thyme, a bay leaf, and spinach.

If you cannot find *nigella seeds in your Indian market or Asian market, just omit them. But if you can find them, it is worth the effort for they have a terrific sweet onion flavor. Mustard seeds are available in the spice section of most supermarkets. Don't bother peeling the fresh ginger. By the time it simmers into the lentils, the peel is undetectable. You can control the spicy heat of the chilies by removing the seeds and inner membranes where capsicum (the compound responsible for the fiery heat) is most concentrated.

Lentils

1 cup split lentils (brown, yellow, black, orange, or any combination)
4 cups water
1 teaspoon minced ginger
1 teaspoon minced garlic
1 teaspoon turmeric
2 small diced fresh green chilies (like jalapenos), stemmed, seeded, white membranes removed
1 teaspoon salt

Onion-Tomato Marmalade

2 tablespoons vegetable oil
1 onion sliced

1 teaspoon mustard seed
½ teaspoon black onion seed (nigella seeds) *optional
3 dried red chilies (like chiles japones or chiles arbol)
1 tomato, sliced

Garnish

Plain yogurt (whole-milk is preferred)
1 tablespoon chopped cilantro
1-2 fresh green chilies, seeded and sliced
1 tablespoon chopped fresh mint

Boil Lentils

Rinse the lentils and pick out any rocks or debris. Boil the lentils in the water with the ginger, garlic, salt, turmeric, and chopped green chilies for 15-20 minutes or until soft. If desired, mash the lentil mixture down. The consistency of the mashed lentils should be similar to soft mashed potatoes. If the mixture looks dry, add more water. Adjust seasoning with more salt if necessary.

Prepare marmalade

Heat the oil on medium and fry the onion with the mustard, onion seeds, and dried red chilies for 2 minutes. Add tomato and cook on low for another 5 minutes, stirring occasionally, until mixture is browned, sweet, and savory.

Assemble the Lentils

Spoon the onion-tomato marmalade over the lentils and top with a dollop of plain yogurt. Garnish with fresh cilantro, green chilies, and mint. This dish is excellent with steamed basmati rice.

Tomato, Kale, & White Bean Stew with Sage

Serves 6

This Tuscan vegetarian dish is the perfect way to use up late-summer herbs, tomatoes, kale, onions, and zucchini. In a pinch, canned tomatoes will do. With bold flavors and a rich stew texture, it screams "comfort food" when the weather turns colder. Serve it with crusty multi-grain bread topped with Parmesan cheese for a complete meal.

*Kale is a member of the cruciferous family along with broccoli, cauliflower, and cabbage. It is dark green with rather tough leaves. Although kale has a bitter taste and is used more for buffet garnish than for eating, it happens to claim the prize as one of the most nutritious vegetables on the planet. This is a good way to enjoy it. Baby kale is more tender than the larger, mature leaves and takes less time to cook. Remove the tough center stalk before chopping leaves.

3-4 tablespoons olive oil
1 small onion, diced
3 pounds very ripe tomatoes, chopped (about 4 cups)
2 cloves garlic, finely diced
2 (15 ounce) cans white beans (Cannelini, Great Northern, etc.), drain and rinse one can
3 cups baby kale*, chopped (or use spinach)
2 cups zucchini, chopped or shredded
4-5 large fresh sage leaves, chopped or 1 teaspoon dried
¼ cup chopped flat-leaf Italian parsley (not curly parsley) or 1 teaspoon dried
a pinch crushed red pepper flakes
salt and pepper to taste
parmesan cheese for garnish

Heat oil in a large heavy-bottomed pot on medium heat. Add onion and sauté for a minute. Add garlic and cook for only 30 seconds stirring constantly. Add tomatoes with their juices all at once. Add the drained can of beans and then dump in the second can with its juices. Stir to incorporate. Add kale, zucchini, sage, and crushed red pepper flakes. Adjust seasoning with salt and pepper. It may require a lot of salt—beans are funny that way.

Simmer on medium low for at least ½ hour, stirring occasionally. If mixture seems dry, add water and a bit of olive oil.

Serve with grated parmesan cheese.

Meatless Garden Burgers

Makes about 36 (4 inch) patties

Have you ever thought, "I bet I could make that"? This recipe came from reading the ingredients on the box of a very tasty commercial vegetable burger and deciding to make my own version. According to the judges at my house, the homemade burgers win! Believe it or not, these vegetarian babies taste better to my kids than burgers made from ground beef. They freeze well and can go directly from freezer to frying pan.

Vegans take heart: To make these without the cheese and eggs, substitute 4 additional cups cooked barley (al dente) and ¼ cup olive oil, or use soy cheese.

*Tip: For ease, cook the brown rice and barley together in a rice cooker using the same ratio of grain-to-water as you normally would for rice alone (two-to-one). Use the chopping blade of a food processor for mincing the mushrooms, onion, bell pepper, and sun-dried tomatoes.

8 cups cooked brown rice
1 cup pearl barley

½ cup bulger wheat
24 ounces fresh white mushrooms, brushed for dirt
½ medium onion, coarsely chopped
2 tablespoons green or red bell pepper, finely minced
2 tablespoons sun-dried tomatoes, reconstituted until soft in ½ cup boiling water, drained
2 ounces mozzarella cheese, shredded
1 ounce cheddar cheese, shredded
1 ounce parmesan cheese, shredded
3 cups old-fashioned oatmeal, uncooked
1 ½ teaspoons garlic powder
1 tablespoon dried parsley flakes
2 tablespoons lemon juice or 1 teaspoon lemon pepper
1 teaspoon turmeric (for color)
2 eggs, whisked in a small bowl with a fork
salt and pepper to taste
olive oil for frying

Prep Ingredients

Cook brown rice and barley in a rice cooker according to manufacturer's directions with water and 1 teaspoon salt. Transfer to a very large bowl to cool. Place bulgar wheat in a small bowl and pour 1 cup boiling water over top. Allow wheat to soak until rice and barley are cool enough to handle. Drain bulgar and add to barley and brown rice. In a food processor, pulse mushrooms until coarsely chopped, scraping bowl periodically. Add onions, peppers, and sun-dried tomatoes. Continue to process until mixture is finely minced, but not pureed. It should have some coarse texture. Using large paper towels, squeeze as much moisture as possible from the mushroom mixture. Add to rice mixture in large bowl.

Make Patties

Preheat oven to 375 degrees. Add all remaining ingredients to rice mixture. Mix well. Season generously with salt and pepper to taste. Using a wide spoon, scoop ½ cup handfuls of mixture into your hands. Pressing firmly, form into balls approximately the size of a large egg. Compress slightly and flatten into 4 inch patties of uniform ¼ inch thickness. Place on a parchment-lined baking sheet until all the patties are formed.

Bake sheets of burgers for 20 minutes, until cheese starts to ooze and patties start to brown. Cool completely on parchment. Bag patties and store in freezer until ready to use. Garden burgers can be stored in a freezer for up to one month.

To Serve

Heat a little olive oil in a large frying pan. Fry patties in batches, leaving space between them so patties will brown. When golden crisp on one side, flip garden burgers onto the other side. Serve patties on toast or buns with mayonnaise, ketchup, lettuce, and tomato.

Winter Vegetable Stew over Couscous

Makes about 10 servings

This North African-inspired dish serves a crowd. Prepare the couscous while the vegetable mixture simmers. Try serving with harissa, a Tunisian hot sauce found in Middle Eastern markets and large grocery stores. Or, use leftover harissa sauce from Moroccan Lamb recipe on page .

*Swiss chard has big, wide dimpled green leaves, with a red or white center stalk. Unlike kale, chard is tender and cooks quickly. Spinach makes a good substitute.

11 ½ cups water, divided into 10 cups and 1 ½ cups

4 cups vertically sliced onion

2 cups thinly sliced leek

1 ½ cups (½ inch thick) sliced carrot

3 cups (1 inch) cubed peeled turnips—about 1 pound

1 bay leaf

4 cups (1 inch) cubed, peeled butternut squash—about 1 ½ pounds

1 teaspoon ground cumin

½ teaspoon ground red pepper (cayenne)

½ teaspoon ground cinnamon

pinch of saffron (about ⅛ teaspoon)

4 garlic cloves, minced

1 (15 ½ ounce) can chickpeas (garbanzo beans), rinsed and drained

6 cups chopped Swiss chard* (about 12 ounces)

½ cup chopped cilantro

2 ½ teaspoons salt, divided into 2 teaspoons and a ½ teaspoon

½ teaspoon freshly ground black pepper

2 tablespoons fresh lemon juice

3 cups uncooked couscous

2 tablespoons extra virgin olive oil

1½ cups (6 ounces) crumbled goat or feta cheese (optional)

1 ½ cups fried almonds (optional)

Combine 10 cups water and the next 5 ingredients in a large heavy pot; bring to a boil. Cover, reduce heat, and simmer 30 minutes. Remove 2 cups cooking liquid; set aside. Add squash and next 6 ingredients to onion mixture. Simmer 15 minutes or until squash is tender. Stir in chard, cilantro, 2 teaspoons salt, and black pepper; cook 5 minutes or until chard wilts. Stir in lemon juice. Discard bay leaf.

Place couscous in a large lidded pan or bowl. Combine reserved cooking liquid and remaining 1½ cups water in a small saucepan; bring to a boil. Stir in remaining ½ teaspoon salt and oil. Pour boiling water mixture over couscous; stir well to combine. Cover tightly and let stand 20 minutes or until liquid is absorbed. Fluff couscous with a fork. Serve vegetable mixture over couscous. Top with crumbled cheese and/or fried almonds.

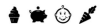

Zucchini-Corn Fritters with Basil Mayonnaise

Makes 20 (3 inch) patties

When zucchini the size of Volkswagons appear anonymously on your doorstep during the last days of summer, turn them into this delicious vegetarian dish. These fritters are the perfect way to use up squash along with other prolific garden vegetables like corn, onions, tomatoes, peppers, and basil. With the aid of a food processor, zucchini takes only seconds to shred. While the fritters are chilling, make the basil mayonnaise.

This recipe calls for serving fritters as part of an assembled salad. However, they are equally good on a toasted bun with a dollop of basil mayonnaise—recipe follows.

2 pounds zucchini squash, or other similar variety, such as yellow crookneck squash
2 cups corn kernels, fresh or canned, drained
½ cup green pepper, cut into 1 inch chunks
½ cup onion, cut into 1 inch chunks
2 eggs
salt and pepper to taste
½ cup flour
⅛ teaspoon cayenne pepper
3-4 cups cracker crumbs or panko bread crumbs (crunchy Japanese bread crumbs)
Olive oil for frying
Ripe tomato, sliced into wheels
Basil mayonnaise (recipe follows)
Mixed salad greens

Make Filling

Use processor to shred zucchini, onion, and green pepper. In a large bowl, combine zucchini, onion, green pepper, and corn. Salt and pepper to taste. Mix in flour and cayenne pepper. In a small bowl, whisk eggs with a fork until blended. Pour egg over vegetable mixture and mix well.

Shape Patties

Line two baking sheets with parchment paper and set aside. Place cracker crumbs in a wide shallow bowl. Drop zucchini mixture by ¼ cupfuls into the center of crumbs. Using hands, scoop crumbs under and around wet filling, pressing to adhere, shaping patties into approximately 3 inches wide and no more than a ½ inch thick. Place crumb-coated patties on prepared parchment-lined baking sheets. When sheet is full, freeze until patties are firm.

Cook Fritters

Preheat oven to 425 degrees. Heat 3 tablespoons olive oil in two large frying pans until hot, but not smoking. Add patties, leaving room between so they do not touch. When brown, flip patties onto other side. Transfer browned patties back to parchment-lined sheets. Wipe out fry pans between batches and replace with fresh oil until all patties are browned. Bake sheets of browned fritters in preheated oven 20 minutes until crisp and brown.

Assemble

Toss mixed greens with some basil mayonnaise. Arrange dressed greens on individual serving plates. Top with a hot fritter, a slice of fresh ripe tomato, and a dollop of basil mayonnaise. Serve.

*Note: Extra fritters can be frozen on baking sheet, uncooked, and then transferred to plastic freezer bags. Fritters keep for one month in freezer.

Basil Mayonnaise

Yield: 1 cup

Try basil mayonnaise as a salad dressing by thinning with a little water until proper consistency
1 cup mayonnaise
¼ cup basil leaves, packed

Finely chop basil until it starts to release juices. Quickly stir into mayonnaise so basil does not oxidize (brown). Refrigerate for at least 20 minutes. Keeps in refrigerator up to ten days.

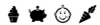

Fresh Egg Raviolis with Ricotta Cheese

Serves 8 entrée portions

You gotta be kidding! Who makes their own pasta? Actually, this labor of love is fun and takes less time than reading this recipe all the way through; and if you have never felt the velvety texture of hand-made pasta as it feeds through your fingers, you might not know what you are missing. Making pasta is a tactile treat. Without question, fresh pasta is superior in taste and mouth-feel compared to dried commercial products. Quanta bella!

Use this dough recipe for any pasta shape. If you don't have an old-fashioned pasta-rolling machine, use a rolling pin. My son turns the crank till his arm aches—I like to think of it as sweat equity.

Remember to give yourself enough time for the pasta dough to rest in the refrigerator. Use fresh flour and eggs because you will taste the difference. I serve these simple cheese raviolis with a sauce of pureed butternut squash simmered with coconut milk and sage. However, browned butter is a perfect simple sauce for these toothsome raviolis. Classic and simple.

Pasta
3 cups unbleached all-purpose flour
5 large eggs, beaten
½ teaspoon salt
1 tablespoon extra-virgin olive oil
water, add a teaspoon at a time

Filling
2-3 cups ricotta cheese
2 eggs whites, beaten until barely frothy

Prepare the pasta:
Place all pasta ingredients except water in a large standing mixer bowl with dough hook attachment. On low speed, combine ingredients. Increase speed and add water one teaspoon at a time until dough is soft but not sticky. When dough forms a ball and pulls away from the sides of the bowl (about 5 minutes) remove dough from bowl and wrap completely in plastic wrap. Dust with flour if dough is too sticky to pull out of the bowl. Allow dough ball to rest in the refrigerator for at least 30 minutes (or overnight).

Roll out pasta sheets:

Divide dough into six equal pieces. Keep dough pieces refrigerated in plastic wrap until ready to use. Dust dough with flour and slightly flatten one edge. Use flour sparingly because incorporating too much flour into the dough will make it tough. With pasta roller on widest setting, roll dough through the rollers to approximately ⅛ inch thickness.

Run pasta through rollers several times to make a sheet of uniform thickness. Adjust the rollers to the next smaller setting and roll dough through several more times. Continue reducing the roller settings and rolling dough until a long uniform sheet is formed. Dust with a little more flour if sheets become too sticky to handle. Stop when rolling on the second-to-last setting (about ¹⁄₁₆ inch thickness). Pasta sheets should not be paper-thin. If dough becomes too long to manage, cut it in half to achieve sheets approximately 5 inches wide and 18 inches long. Do not worry if sheets are not exact rectangles.

Make Raviolis:
On a floured surface, lay out half of pasta sheets. Using a pasta cutter, pizza cutter, or sharp knife, trim edges to make sheets uniform in width. Mound teaspoonfuls of ricotta cheese in two rows at 3 inch intervals along the length of the pasta strip. Using a pastry brush, paint around and between raviolis with egg white. Lay another strip of pasta over the top. Press around filling to adhere top sheet to bottom, leaving space around cheese for expansion. Cut between cheese mounds to make uniform squares of ravioli. Repeat with remaining pasta strips. Allow raviolis to rest on lightly flour-dusted baking sheets until ready to cook. Sheets can be wrapped with plastic and refrigerated or frozen until ready to cook.

Cook Pasta:
Bring six quarts of salted water to boil in a large stock-pot. Working in batches, cook half of raviolis at a time, stirring occasionally. Fresh pasta takes only 2-3 minutes to cook and floats to the top when done. Taste to check if pasta is done. When pasta is al dente, remove with a slotted spoon to a colander. Cook remaining raviolis. Serve immediately with your favorite sauce. Or, simply drizzle melted butter over raviolis and serve.

Turkey Entrees

Stuffed Cabbage

Serves 8

After wolfing down these savory little purses, my kids proclaimed, "I like cabbage."

Upon returning from a church service mission in Romania, my dear friend Jeanne Engberson shared with me her recipe for Romanian stuffed cabbage. I fused her recipe with another variation of stuffed cabbage I had previously enjoyed in Germany. The German stuffed cabbage was prepared for me by excellent Polish cooks, which makes this recipe a Roma-Germa-Pol-American amalgamation of this venerable dish. It is a veritable United Nations of stuffed Cabbage and a great way to use up leftover rice!

2 (8 ounce) cans plain tomato sauce
1 large head cabbage
2 pounds ground turkey
½ cup onion, finely chopped
½ cup carrot, finely chopped
¼ cup green chilies (seeds and membrane removed) or green pepper, finely chopped
1 teaspoon fresh ginger, finely minced
1 tablespoon dried parsley
1 tablespoon dried dill leaf
1 ½ cups cooked brown or white rice, cooled
2 teaspoons salt
fresh ground pepper
olive oil for preparing pan
plain yogurt or sour cream (optional)

Grease 9 x 13 inch casserole dish with olive oil. Pour one of the 8 ounce cans of tomato sauce over bottom of casserole and set aside. Preheat oven to 350 degrees.

Core cabbage and separate outer two-thirds of leaves from the compact inner leaves, keeping large leaves intact for filling. Finely chop remaining inner third of cabbage (the leaves that will not separate), and set aside.

In a large sauté pan, brown ground turkey until cooked through. Transfer turkey to a large mixing bowl, reserving oil and juices in pan. In same pan on medium heat, sauté onion, carrot, chili, and ginger. Stir until vegetables start to soften. Add vegetables to the large bowl with the turkey. Season mixture with parsley, dill, salt, and pepper. Stir to combine. Adjust seasonings to taste. Add rice and reserved chopped cabbage. Mix well.

Fill cabbage leaves with ½ cup filling. If leaves have cracks or holes, layer several leaves together. Roll up and place in prepared pan, seam side down. Continue filling leaves, arranging them snugly in pan. Spoon any remaining filling between gaps in pan. Pour remaining can of tomato sauce down center of rolls. Cover casserole tightly with foil.

Bake in preheated oven 1 hour. Serve with a dollop of plain yogurt or sour cream if desired.

Braised Turkey Legs

Serves 4-6 entrees

This recipe is a variation on the quintessential French dish Coq Au Vin (chicken in wine). Although we don't consider turkey a typical French food, it is surprisingly common in the French countryside. This kind of slow-cooked comfort food has long been a mainstay in rural France and is consistent with the original "peasant food" of medieval Europe.

Spoon tender turkey and rich braising liquid over mashed potatoes or noodles. To make your own homemade noodles use the ravioli pasta recipe on page and cut noodles into 1 inch wide strips to make traditional paparadelle or tagliatelle.

*Demi-glacé (pronounced demi-gloss) is a reduced sauce made from beef stock, shallots, and red wine. The concentrated flavors add dimension to this dish. Demi-glacé can be purchased in small quantities at gourmet markets and some supermarkets.

4 turkey legs or 3 thighs with skin (about 2-3 pounds)
3 tablespoons butter, olive oil, or bacon grease (or a combination of all three) divided into 2 tablespoons and 1 tablespoon

¾ cup white onion, chopped or 1 cup pearl onions, peeled

2 carrots, chopped

3 shallots, minced (about ¼ cup chopped), located in the produce section with garlic and onion

2 garlic cloves, minced

2 tablespoons tomato paste

3 tablespoons flour

2 tablespoons parsley, minced

2 bay leaves

2 teaspoons fresh thyme leaves

1 ½ cup dry red wine or sherry (about ¼ of a bottle) *or* beef stock

½ cup demi-glacé* or 1 tablespoon concentrated beef paste

1 tablespoon Dijon mustard

1 tablespoon brandy, *or* cider vinegar

½ cup chicken stock or hot water

½ pound fresh mushrooms, left whole if small or halved if large

fresh ground pepper and salt

Heat 2 tablespoons butter and/or oil in large heavy pot. Sprinkle poultry with salt and fresh ground pepper. Brown turkey pieces thoroughly. They will smoke. Remove from pot. Using same pot without wiping it out, add remaining 1 tablespoon fat and sauté vegetables until lightly browned. Stir flour into vegetables. Add wine and stir pot, scraping up browned bits. When the wine is mostly absorbed, stir in herbs, brandy, demi-glacé, and Dijon mustard. Return turkey to the vegetable pot, adding any accumulated juices. Paint turkey pieces with tomato paste to evenly coat. Add chicken stock or hot water, increasing to one cup if mixture looks dry. Cover and simmer over low heat until done, about 1 hour, and up to 2 hours. Ten minutes before serving, add mushrooms. Correct the seasoning and serve the turkey and vegetables over noodles or potatoes. Garnish with fresh herbs.

Variations: You can successfully substitute chicken legs or beef short ribs for the turkey. The most traditional version of this dish includes minced salt pork or pancetta in the initial browning of the turkey, instead of bacon grease. The tomato paste substitutes for chicken blood that traditionally would have been used for color, flavor, and thickening. If you like extra sauce, increase the wine to 2 cups. Other fresh vegetables may be added such as zucchini, potatoes, parsnips, celery, peas, etc.

Other Meats

Moroccan Roasted Lamb With Harissa Sauce

Serves 8

This recipe is based on the spit-roasted lamb of Morocco and is my all-time favorite lamb preparation. Because most of us don't have a backyard pit of hot coals, this convenient version works in the oven. Start with a very hot oven and then lower the heat, basting diligently with pan juices every fifteen minutes. The results are a buttery-tender inside and a deliciously crunchy outside. This scaled-down version is made with boneless leg of lamb, but bone-in or even a full ten-pound forequarter is closer to the authentic Moroccan preparation. Use what you can find and enjoy every hot mouthful.

3 ½ pounds boneless leg of lamb (for lamb with the bone-in, use about 5-6 pounds)
2 tablespoons butter
2 cloves garlic, peeled and mashed
salt and pepper to taste
1 teaspoon ground cumin
1 teaspoon sweet paprika
1 tablespoon ground coriander seed (found in the spice section of your supermarket)
twine or skewers

Preheat oven to 475 degrees. In a small bowl, combine butter, garlic, salt and pepper, cumin, paprika, and coriander. On work surface, lay out lamb, fat side up. Trim fat to ½ inch thick. Make long ½ inch deep slits down the layer of top fat. Spread seasoned butter over the whole lamb, rubbing into slits. Roll lamb back up into a uniform roast and secure with twine or skewers. Place lamb in a large roasting pan and allow it to rest for ten minutes. Roast lamb in oven for fifteen minutes and then turn down oven to 350 degrees. Baste frequently with pan juices. Continue roasting until lamb is tender and internal thermometer reads 170 degrees. Allow meat to rest ten minutes before digging in. Meat should still be slightly pink. Reserve pan drippings for Harissa Sauce (see following recipe). Slice lamb and serve with couscous and sauce.

Harissa Sauce

Use the pan drippings from the roasted lamb to make this terrific savory sauce. It takes the concept of "au jus" to a whole new level.

1 can low-salt beef broth
1 teaspoon sambal oelek (Indonesian chili sauce called *Sriracha*—found in the Asian section of most supermarkets), or use any hot sauce
1 tablespoon lemon juice
1-2 tablespoons olive oil
pinch of ground cumin, to taste
1 tablespoon parsley, finely chopped
1 tablespoon cilantro, finely chopped

Remove lamb from roasting pan. Heat pan drippings over medium high heat. Add enough beef broth to drippings to yield at least one cup of liquid. Whisk in all other ingredients and heat to simmer. Pour sauce into a small serving bowl and spoon over hot slices of Moroccan Lamb. Pass sauce separately.

Wild Mushroom & Prosciutto Pizza

Makes two ten-inch pizzas

This is a great master recipe for pizza crust. However, in a pinch, feel free to use a purchased pre-cooked crust.

For Crust:
1 envelope active dry yeast
1 ½ cups warm water, separated
salt
1 tablespoon extra-virgin olive oil, plus extra for oiling baking sheets
3 ½ cups bread flour (approximately)

In a large mixing bowl of a standing mixer, stir yeast and ½ cup warm water. Allow yeast mixture to proof for about ten minutes. The yeast mixture will begin to bubble and foam.

Add the remaining warm water, a pinch of salt, and the olive oil. Using the dough hook attachment, mix in flour one cup at a time on low speed. It should be moist but not sticky. Continue to knead on medium speed for about two more minutes until dough has a smooth velvety feel. (This can be done by hand if you don't have a standing mixer.)

Form dough into a large ball and transfer to an oiled bowl. Cover with plastic wrap and allow dough to rise in a warm place for about one hour.

When dough has risen and is double in size, punch it down and divide dough into two halves. Refrigerate, freeze, or proceed with pizza recipe.

Invert two baking sheets and using a pastry brush paint a large circle on the back with olive oil—this is your baking surface. Sprinkle the oiled area with cornmeal. Using floured hands and dusting dough lightly with flour, stretch out each half into 10 inch diameter circles. Crusts should be thin. Don't worry if there are holes in dough—just stretch to patch. Place pizza circles on backs of prepared baking sheets. Cover and allow dough to rest 30 minutes. Preheat oven to 450 degrees. Proceed with toppings and bake.

For Mushroom Topping:
2 tablespoons extra-virgin olive oil
16 ounces fresh sliced mushrooms (cremini, shitake, porcini, oyster, or plain-old button mushrooms)
½ cup finely chopped shallots
2 garlic cloves, minced
2 teaspoons chopped fresh thyme
1 ½ tablespoons balsamic, or sherry vinegar
6 ounces prosciutto cut in strips (thinly sliced dry-cured ham) *or* any good-quality ham
1 cup fontina cheese, shredded, *or* substitute gouda, Swiss, farmer cheese, or mozzarella

Heat oil in a large skillet over medium heat. Sauté mushrooms and shallots until mushrooms are tender. Add garlic and thyme; sauté 1 minute. Stir in vinegar. Remove from heat.

Spread mushroom mixture on top of dough. Arrange prosciutto and cheese on top of mushrooms. Place pan in the bottom of a 450 degree oven and bake for 12-15 minutes, until crust is done and slightly browned at the edges. Serve.

Other Stuff

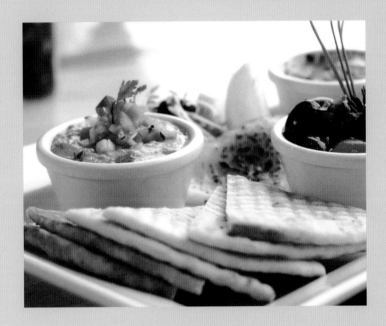

Hummus, page 221

Chinese Dumplings With Lamb, Carrot, & Chive

Makes 60 dumplings

Two amazing Chinese friends showed me how to make authentic dumplings during a summer evening in my kitchen, which resulted in this recipe for toothsome little pillows, beautifully formed and irresistibly tasty. Don't make the mistake of assuming you will eat only one. In China, a whole tray of dumplings dipped in black vinegar and chili oil makes a typical breakfast.

The two keys to great dumplings: finely mince all the filling ingredients and avoid the tendency to over-fill the wrappers (too much filling makes the dumplings difficult to seal).

For a vegetarian variation, omit the lamb and chives to make delicious Carrot-Ginger Dumplings.

Filling
1 cup white onion, finely diced
1 pound lamb, well-ground
2 cups grated and then finely chopped carrots
3-4 tablespoons fresh grated ginger
3-4 tablespoons finely chopped fresh chives
1 egg, lightly beaten
1 ½ tablespoons soy sauce
salt to taste
2 tablespoons olive or peanut oil
1 package fresh round won ton or dumpling wrappers (about 60)
small bowl of water

Sauce
1 tablespoon soy sauce
1 tablespoon Chinese black vinegar, available at Asian markets
1 teaspoon minced garlic
1 heaping teaspoon sambal (Indonesian chili paste found in the Asian aisle of most supermarkets)
1 tablespoon scallion, chopped fine

Make lamb filling:
Wrap chopped onion in several layers of paper towels and squeeze between hands to extract as much moisture as possible. Transfer onion to a medium size mixing bowl. Add next four

ingredients and stir well to combine. Add egg, soy sauce, salt, and peanut oil. Using hands, mix very well.

Assemble dumplings:

Place one teaspoon of filling in the center of a dumpling wrapper. Dip finger in water and wet outer edge of wrapper around filling. Cupping the dumpling in one hand, use the other hand to pinch top edge closed, making pleats every ¼ inch or so. With cupping hand, try to shape a fat rounded bottom with a semi-circle of small pleats around the top, like a crown. Seal as you go so no filling escapes during cooking. Deflate any air pockets as you press the edges together. Place dumplings on parchment lined baking sheets and press bottom slightly to flatten so dumpling will stand upright without rolling over. Continue until all dumplings are filled. This fun project can occupy many hands in the kitchen at once.

In a large pot, heat water to almost boiling. Simmer dumplings until they rise to the top of the pot. Test a dumpling by slicing open. They are done when lamb is opaque and dumpling wrapper is tender but still firm.

Make dipping sauce:

Stir together sauce ingredients. Adjust soy sauce to taste. Serve hot dumplings immediately with dipping sauce.

Eggplant-Garlic Spread

Makes 2 cups

In the South of France, this is called eggplant "caviar." It tastes fantastic spread on crusty bread and packs well as a picnic appetizer. It gets better with age, so feel free to make it several days in advance.

1 cup Roma tomatoes, peeled, seeded, and chopped
¼ teaspoon salt
2 pounds eggplant

4 tablespoons plus 1 teaspoon olive oil
½ cup minced onion
2 garlic cloves, minced
4 teaspoons balsamic or red wine vinegar
freshly ground black pepper

Preheat oven to 425 degrees. Place cut tomatoes in a plastic strainer set over a bowl. Sprinkle tomatoes with ¼ teaspoon salt and allow them to drain for 20 minutes.

Split each eggplant in half lengthwise. Drizzle 1 teaspoon oil over the cut tops. Place cut-side down in a baking dish with ½ cup water and bake for 45 minutes until tender, turning them over after 20 minutes. Add more water if necessary. Set aside to cool. Scoop out the flesh of the eggplants with a spoon. Discard eggplant skins.

In a processor, puree the eggplant pulp, drained tomatoes, onion, garlic, remaining oil, vinegar, and ½ teaspoon salt and pepper until smooth. Taste for salt and if necessary, correct seasoning. Cover and chill for a day to develop flavors. Keeps for two weeks in the refrigerator.

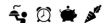

Roasted Asparagus with Almonds, Grapes, & Balsamic Glaze

Serves 8

When selecting asparagus, look for firm, tightly closed tops and firm stems that have been kept upright in a shallow pan of fresh water. Asparagus stalks continue to "drink" after they are cut.

2 pounds fresh asparagus washed and trimmed to remove tough ends
olive oil
1-2 tablespoons balsamic vinegar
salt and pepper to taste
1 cup red seedless grapes, cut in half to release juices when baking
¼ cup sliced almonds

Preheat oven to 375 degrees. On a parchment-lined baking sheet, lay out asparagus spears in a single layer. Drizzle with olive oil and balsamic vinegar. Use a pastry brush to coat asparagus evenly. Season with salt and pepper. Distribute grapes and almonds over asparagus. Roast for 5-10 minutes until crisp tender. Serve immediately.

Quinoa-Walnut Pilaf With Butternut
Squash & Caramelized Onions

Serves 4-6

Quinoa is an ancient grain with a spiral shape and tiny kernels. It has a pleasant nutty flavor and cooks up similar to rice. Quinoa can be enjoyed hot as a side dish or in cold salads.

Toast walnut halves by placing on a baking sheet in a preheated 375 degree oven for approximately 10 minutes, until fragrant and beginning to brown.

Use a standard potato peeler to remove the peel from butternut squash.

2 cups dry quinoa*
2 tablespoons plus 1 teaspoon oil, divided
3 tablespoons butter, divided into 2 tablespoons and 1 tablespoon
½ large onion, cut into ½ inch dice
1 teaspoon honey
1 cup uncooked butternut squash, *peeled, cut into ½ inch dice
1 cup toasted walnut halves*, coarsely chopped
2 tablespoons fresh sage leaves, chopped
2 large garlic cloves, finely minced
2 jalapeño chilies, stemmed, seeds and ribs removed, finely diced
1 tablespoon dry ground ginger
1 cup tomato juice or V-8, vegetable stock or water
1 cup corn kernels, canned or frozen
1 (9-10 ounce) package prepared fresh spinach leaves
1 avocado, sliced
2 cups drained plain yogurt (preferably whole milk)* see method below

Cook quinoa in 4 cups salted water in a covered pot on the stovetop, or use a rice cooker. Quinoa should absorb all the water and still be firm.

In a large, heavy-bottomed saucepan, melt 1 tablespoon butter with 2 tablespoons oil over medium heat. Add diced onion and honey, and stir to coat with oil. Cook until onions begin to brown and take on a sweet caramel flavor (about 7 minutes). Add diced butternut squash, walnuts, and sage. Continue to cook, stirring occasionally until squash begins to brown but is still firm (another 7 minutes). Add garlic, jalapenos, and ginger and cook for one more minute. Add more oil if pan seems dry. Add liquid and corn, and stir to incorporate any browned bits on the bottom of the pan. This is called de-glazing the pan.

Stir cooked quinoa into vegetables. Season pilaf generously with salt and pepper. Stir in remaining one tablespoon of butter. Keep warm on low heat.

In a large pan, wilt spinach in the remaining teaspoon of oil over medium heat. Place a bed of spinach on each plate. Top with quinoa pilaf, avocado slices, and a dollop of thickened yogurt (or purchased sour cream). Serve

Thickened Yogurt

Why cook with yogurt instead of sour cream? Because it is lower in saturated fat and has a distinctly tangy-rich flavor. Yogurt is also creamier with a smoother mouth-feel than sour cream. If you are short on time, don't bother draining it and just plop a spoonful over anything you would garnish with sour cream.

Method
To thicken yogurt, set a fine mesh strainer over a bowl to catch drips and drain whole or low-fat yogurt in the refrigerator at least an hour and up to one day. Store in an airtight container for up to one week. Use in place of sour cream.

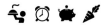

Garden Succotash

Makes 8-10 servings

This is another great way to use summertime vegetables from your garden (or the farmer's market). Onions, peppers, corn, squash, beans, tomatoes, and herbs all come together in this southern side dish. If you prep all the ingredients ahead of time, succotash takes only minutes to cook.

3 tablespoons butter
3 tablespoons olive oil
1 large onion, chopped
1 red bell pepper, cut into ½ inch pieces
½ green bell pepper, cut into ½ inch pieces
1 garlic clove, minced
2 cups fresh corn kernels (cut from about 3 ears) or canned, drained
2 medium-size zucchini, trimmed, cut into ¾ inch pieces
2 medium-size yellow crookneck squash, trimmed, cut into ¾ inch pieces
2 cups cup fresh green beans, cut into 1 inch lengths
4 tablespoons chopped fresh Italian parsley, 1 tablespoon reserved for garnish
1 tablespoon chopped fresh marjoram
1 pound fresh tomatoes, coarsely chopped

Melt butter with oil in heavy large deep skillet over medium-high heat. Add onion, bell peppers, and garlic; sauté until peppers are crisp-tender, about 5 minutes. Add corn, zucchini, yellow squash, and beans; sauté until vegetables are just tender, about 7 minutes longer. Stir in 3 tablespoons parsley and the marjoram. Season to taste with salt and pepper. Transfer succotash to bowl. Top with chopped fresh tomatoes. Sprinkle with remaining 1 tablespoon parsley, salt, and fresh pepper. Serve.

Puree of Fresh Pea Soup with Crème Fraichê

Serves 6

Plan ahead to allow enough time for crème fraichê to thicken overnight. For a super quick meal, use purchased crème fraichê or sour cream for the garnish instead of making your own. The soup itself is a 5-minute recipe—just simmer and puree.

*Créme fraichê is cultured cream—essentially homemade sour cream. It is less thick and goopy than sour cream and has a mild nutty flavor.

3 cups fresh or frozen peas
2 teaspoons fresh chives, snipped fine
5 cups chicken stock or vegetable stock
Fresh mint for garnish
Salt and pepper
Crème Fraichê
Heavy whipping cream
1 tablespoon plain yogurt (with live and active cultures listed on packaging)

Make Soup
Heat first three ingredients in a large pot. When peas are simmering, immerse long-necked hand blender in pot and puree until smooth. Or, puree in a blender in batches. Adjust seasoning with salt and pepper. Serve with a dollop of crème fraichê or sour cream and a sprig of mint.

Make Crème Fraichê
Heat cream just to body temperature (around 98 degrees) in a small saucepan. Check with your finger. When the cream matches your body temperature (neither hot nor cold), take off heat and stir in a tablespoon of plain yogurt. Cover with a clean cloth and allow cream to sit overnight on the counter at room temperature, or at least 8 hours. When it has thickened and taken on a nutty taste, cover tightly and refrigerate. Use within two days.

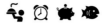

Cauliflower Soup With Chicken, Corn, & Cumin

Serves 6

This soup was inspired by my dear friend Crystelle Francom who helped me test some of the recipes in this book. The pure flavors of cumin and cauliflower are sweetened with the addition of corn. This soup takes less than 10 minutes to get in the pot, and then it simmers unattended for another 20 minutes. Peeled and chopped parsnips make an excellent alternative to cauliflower. For a completely vegetarian soup, substitute edename (soybeans) or tofu for the chicken and replace the chicken broth with vegetable stock.

1 tablespoon olive oil
1 tablespoon cumin seeds, finely ground in spice mill or with mortar and pestle
2 pounds cauliflower, trimmed into 1 inch florets
1 teaspoon white pepper
3 cans low-sodium chicken broth (14 ounces each), or vegetable broth
1 can whole kernel corn with liquid (15.25 ounce)
28 ounces canned cooked chicken chunks with liquid

Heat oil in a large pot on medium heat, until it sizzles when a cumin seed or bread crumb is dropped in it. Add ground cumin and stir 10 seconds until fragrant. Add prepared cauliflower and stir 1 minute more. Add all other ingredients and simmer on low heat until cauliflower is tender and flavors are combined, about 20 minutes. Serve with rye bread and butter.

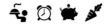

Hummus

....

Makes about 2 ½ cups

I love a do-ahead recipe for entertaining, and this ultra-easy hummus contains all the sunny flavors of the Mediterranean in one bite. Simply pull a bowl of hummus from the refrigerator and get back to your guests. Make it several days ahead to mellow the flavors. To prepare easy pita chips, cut round pita loaves into wedges, brush with butter or olive oil and bake in 375 degree oven 10 minutes, or until chips are crisp and edges start to brown. Serve room temperature hummus with warm chips.

2 (14 ounce) cans garbanzo beans (one can drained)
1 heaping teaspoon minced garlic
5 teaspoons olive oil—or more
2 tablespoons lemon juice (about half of a large lemon)
¼ teaspoon ground cumin
a generous pinch of cayenne pepper
½ teaspoon salt

In a food processor, combine all ingredients and pulse to blend. Continue to process on high until very smooth, scraping occasionally with spatula. Add more olive oil if too thick. Refrigerate. Bring to room temperature before serving. Can be made up to 3 days in advance. Garnish with a drizzle of olive oil and a dusting of paprika. Serve with pita chips.

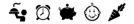

Homemade Blue Cheese Dressing
with Green Goddess and Ranch Dressing Variations

Makes 2 ½ cups

Use equal parts sour cream and buttermilk as a base for a myriad of creamy salad dressings. Be creative.

Green Goddess Variation: Omit bleu cheese, garlic powder, and cayenne. Add chopped capers, walnuts, sweet pickles, and parsley for a delicious Green Goddess dressing.

Ranch Variation: Omit the bleu cheese, cayenne, and garlic powder, and add 2 tablespoons snipped fresh chives.

Blue Cheese Dressing
1 cup sour cream
1 cup buttermilk
½ cup cottage cheese
6 ounces good quality blue cheese (like Maytag, Stilton, or gorgonzola), crumbled
2 tablespoons onion, very finely minced
¼ teaspoon garlic powder
pinch of cayenne pepper
1 teaspoon dried dill
1 teaspoon dried parsley flakes
1 teaspoon salt
Freshly ground black pepper to taste

Whisk all ingredients together. Adjust seasoning with more salt and pepper if desired. Thin with milk if too thick. Chill for at least four hours. Can be kept in a sealed container in the refrigerator for up to a week.

11 quick ways to use zucchini squash

- Cut zucchinis into strips and include them in a platter of crudités (raw vegetable appetizers). Serve with homemade bleu cheese or ranch dressing (see previous recipe).

- Dice them into salads.

- Marinate long zucchini halves in barbecue sauce and grill.

- Chop up any leftover marinated squash into meatloaf. Yum!

- Make coleslaw with shredded zucchini, cabbage, raisins, sunflower seeds, and carrots; toss with lemon-dill vinaigrette or a purchased dressing.

- Make a sauce by pureeing squash in the blender with a little water, garlic, pitted olives, olive oil, and paprika. Pour over pasta or chicken and bake.

- Cut a trench down the center of zucchini halves and stuff with tart apples, celery, and cheddar cheese. Bake until cheese is bubbly.

- Sauté with tomatoes, onions, spinach, and peppers for a quick side dish.

- Make zucchini enchiladas by filling tortillas with chopped zucchini, canned green chilies, scrambled eggs, and cheese.

- Blend a pureed soup from simmered zucchini in chicken stock and garlic. Stir in a dash of Worcestershire sauce and top with chopped avocado and cilantro.

- Stir-fry julienne sticks of zucchini and summer squash in butter and basil. Toss with cooked fettuccini and Parmesan cheese.

- Dip zucchini sticks in an egg wash, then dredge in seasoned bread crumbs. Fry in a pan until crunchy. Serve with marinara sauce for dipping.

Desserts

All desserts can be enjoyed either as a daily treat or as an occasional treat—
according to your body's signals.

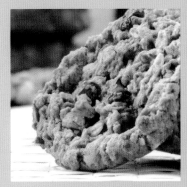

Melanie's Chocolate Chip
Cookies, page 226

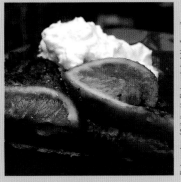

Candied Orange Pecan Pie,
page 229

Photo courtesy of Daily Herald · Photography by Ashley Franscell

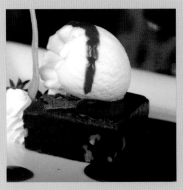

Zucchini-Walnut Brownies with
Ganache Glaze, page 231

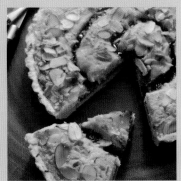

Bakewell Tarts, page 227

Melanie's Chocolate Chip Cookies

Makes approximately 2 dozen big cookies

With a chewy oatmeal texture and chocolate chips, these cookies are outrageously good. This recipe is an adaptation of Melanie Fitts' original cookie recipe. It was given to my sister, who subsequently gave it to my other sister, who finally bequeathed it to me. Hand-me-down recipes taste just as good! Try using good quality chocolate chopped into chunks instead of chocolate chips.

2 sticks unsalted butter
1 cup white sugar
1 cup brown sugar
2 eggs
1 teaspoon vanilla
1 teaspoon baking powder
1 teaspoon baking soda
1 teaspoon salt
½ teaspoon cinnamon
2 cups all-purpose flour (if desired, use half white flour and half whole wheat flour)
2 ½ cups oatmeal
6 ounces chocolate chips (semi-sweet or milk chocolate)
1 cup walnuts, chopped (optional)

Preheat oven to 350 degrees. Cream butter and both sugars until fluffy. Beat in eggs and vanilla until light in color. In a separate large bowl, whisk together baking powder, baking soda, salt, cinnamon, flour, and oatmeal. Add half of dry mixture to wet mixture, stirring just enough to mix together. Add the rest of the dry mixture. Refrain from over-mixing. Add chocolate chips (or chunks) and walnuts, stirring by hand. Dough will be very stiff. Space 1½ inch clumps of dough on a parchment-lined baking sheet, flattening balls a little with the heel of your hand. Bake 10 minutes or just until edges are set. Cool. Store in airtight container in the refrigerator for up to 3 days, or freeze.

Bakewell Tarts

Makes 2 (9-inch) Tarts

After listening to me whine about how difficult it is to find Bakewell tarts in the U.S., my dear English friend promptly came over to my house and, in true Anglican fashion, "just got on with it" and demonstrated how to make them. My sincere thanks to Aimy Kersey for my delightful hands-on cooking class. These traditional English tarts are a particular favorite at tea-time. The buttery almond flavor combined with sweet jam is heady stuff. Feel free to make your own pastry crusts, but this recipe calls for frozen store-bought pie crusts, which work just fine. Other than spreading jam on the bottom of the crust and mixing up the filling in the processor, this recipe is so quick and easy it all but bakes itself.

Ingredients

2 ready-to-bake, frozen pie crusts in 9 inch foil pans

Filling
6 tablespoons jam (raspberry, blackberry, marionberry, or a combination), divided
2 ounces raw almonds (about ⅓ cup)
4 ounces sugar (about ½ cup)
2 ounces flour (about a heaping ⅓ cup)
4 ounces unsalted butter (1 stick)
2 eggs
1 teaspoon almond extract

Preheat oven to 350 degrees. Using back of spoon, spread 3 tablespoons jam uniformly over the bottom of each frozen pie crust. In a food processor, grind almonds with sugar and flour until finely ground. Add butter, eggs, and almond extract and continue to process until mixture is whipped and fluffy. Dividing equally between both tarts, spoon almond mixture over jam, extending all the way to the crust, encasing jam completely.

Bake in the lower third of a preheated oven for about 30 minutes, or until knife comes out clean. If desired, glaze tart after baking by painting it with warmed jam and decorate with sliced almonds. Cool and refrigerate until ready to serve. Can be frozen in pie tin in sealed storage bags for up to 1 month.

Loaded Banana Cookies

Makes about 40 cookies

You could label these cookies "healthy," but somehow that classification diminishes the appeal of this, or any cookie. They are naturally delicious and full of healthy things, butter aside. And in defense of butter, if you are going to eat a cookie, shouldn't it taste good? Let's just call them "loaded" and leave it at that.

*Whole- wheat pastry flour is available in the bulk-food bins of some supermarkets and most health food stores.

¾ cup unsalted butter
1 cup brown sugar
1 egg
1 cup mashed banana (about 2 large ripe bananas)
2 cups whole-wheat pastry flour * (or regular whole wheat flour)
¾ cup cornmeal
½ cup old-fashioned rolled oats
1 teaspoon baking soda
¾ teaspoon salt
1 teaspoon cinnamon
½ teaspoon ground nutmeg
½ teaspoon ground cloves
1-2 cups dried fruit, chopped (apricot, fig, prune, cherry, etc.)
1 cup walnuts, chopped
1-1½ cups chocolate chips (optional)

Preheat oven to 375 degrees, and line baking sheets with parchment paper.

Beat butter and sugar well. Add egg and beat till fluffy. Beat in mashed banana. Whisk together dry ingredients and add to butter mixture in two additions. Stir in fruits, nuts, and chocolate chips. Drop by tablespoon onto cookie sheets. Bake 10-12 minutes.

Candied Orange Pecan Pie

Serves 8-10

*To toast pecans, place on a baking sheet in a 375 degree oven for about 10 minutes, until fragrant and beginning to brown.

Candied Oranges
2 firm seedless oranges (Valencia are good)
2 cups water
1 cup sugar

Crust
1 ¼ cups all purpose flour
½ tablespoon sugar
½ teaspoon salt
1 teaspoon orange zest, chopped fine
½ cup (1 stick) chilled unsalted butter, cut into ½ inch cubes
4 tablespoons (or more) ice water

Filling
1 cup golden brown sugar
1 cup light corn syrup
¼ cup unsalted butter, melted
3 large eggs
1 teaspoon grated orange peel
1 tablespoon orange juice concentrate
1 teaspoon vanilla extract
¼ teaspoon salt
2 cups pecan halves (about 9 ½ ounces), toasted*

Make Crust:
Blend flour, sugar, salt, and orange zest in processor. Add butter and pulse until coarse meal forms. Add 4 tablespoons ice water. Using short pulses, process just until moist clumps form, adding more water if necessary. Gather dough into ball; flatten into disk. Wrap in plastic; refrigerate 1 hour. Can be made 2 days ahead. Keep chilled. Soften slightly at room temperature before rolling. Makes one 9 inch crust

Make Candied Oranges:

In a small pot, over medium heat, stir water and sugar until sugar dissolves. Slice oranges into ⅛ inch wheels, discarding ends. Slice each wheel in half to make half-moons. Add orange slices to sugar syrup and stir gently to submerge. Simmer on medium low heat for at least ½ hour. Remove pot from heat and cool completely in syrup. Drain well before using (reserve syrup for other uses).

Make Pie:

Roll out dough on floured surface to a 13 inch round. Transfer to a 9 inch deep-dish glass pie dish. Trim overhang to ½ inch. Fold overhang under; crimp edges decoratively. Refrigerate 1 hour.

Preheat oven to 375 degrees. Line pie crust with foil and fill with weights (pie weights or dried beans—to prevent crust from puffing up). Bake crust until edges begin to brown and crust is set, about 17 minutes. Remove foil and weights. Bake another 5 minutes until crust is golden brown. Remove from oven and maintain oven temperature.

Whisk brown sugar, corn syrup, melted butter, orange peel, orange juice concentrate, salt, and vanilla extract in a large bowl. Whisk in eggs, one at a time. Stir in toasted pecans. Pour filling into prepared crust. Top with 8-10 candied orange pieces (arranged so each slice will have an orange piece). Bake pie until edges puff and center is just set, about 50 minutes. Cool pie on rack at least 1 hour. Refrigerate. Can be made one day in advance.

Zucchini-Walnut Brownies With Ganache Glaze

Makes one 9 x 13 pan

* Ganache is the rich combination of chocolate melted together with cream. Traditionally used as truffle filling, ganache can be made softer, for sauces and garnish; or firmer, for use in candy and molds, simply by adjusting how much cream is used. After cooling, try whipping it to a piping consistency for fancy cake decorating.

No one in my family suspects zucchini is hidden inside these moist brownies. They are nice and chocolaty, but not overwhelmingly rich. Try using light olive oil for additional health benefits. By my estimation, the anti-oxidant combination of zucchini, nuts, dark chocolate, and olive oil practically make this health food. The glaze is optional, but so very good I highly recommend it.

2 cups zucchini, finely grated
½ cup oil
1 ½ cups sugar
2 teaspoons vanilla
2 cups flour
¼ cup cocoa
1 ½ teaspoons baking soda
1 teaspoon salt
1 cup chopped walnuts (optional)
6 ounces good quality dark chocolate
½ cup cream

Preheat oven to 350 degrees. In a large bowl, mix zucchini, oil, sugar and vanilla. In a medium bowl, whisk together dry ingredients. Add dry ingredients to wet mixture. Mix until just combined. Gently stir in nuts. Spray a 9 x 13 inch pan with cooking spray. Spread batter into pan. Bake for 20-30 minutes. Cool.

In a small bowl set over (not in) simmering water, melt chocolate and cream together, stirring frequently. Pour melted ganache over brownies and spread to edges of pan. Refrigerate to set icing. Cut into squares and serve. For neat, even slices try dipping a thin knife blade in very hot water and wiping dry between each cut.

Recipe Index

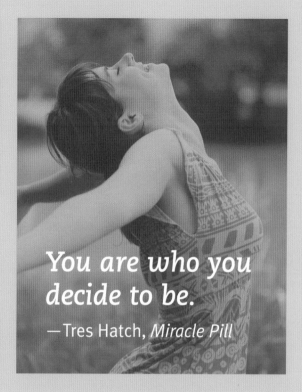

The Power of Today

No one on earth can change yesterday. Just take care of today.

—Tres Hatch, *Miracle Pill*

You are who you decide to be.

—Tres Hatch, *Miracle Pill*

It is not our occasional treats that define our bodies—it is our regular food choices that determine how we look and feel.

—Tres Hatch, *Miracle Pill*

Quick weight loss is the antithesis of permanent weight loss.

—Tres Hatch, *Miracle Pill*

Marketing campaigns promise to do for us that which we can only do for ourselves.

—Tres Hatch, *Miracle Pill*

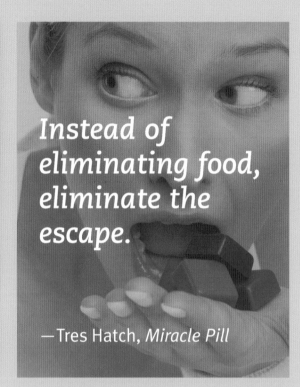

Instead of eliminating food, eliminate the escape.

—Tres Hatch, *Miracle Pill*

Universal laws dictate when you give nothing, you get nothing.

—Tres Hatch, *Miracle Pill*

Even if you only have 10 minutes today, use that precious time to exercise.

—Tres Hatch, *Miracle Pill*

Remove this page and post it where you will see it daily.

Remove this page and post it where you will see it daily.

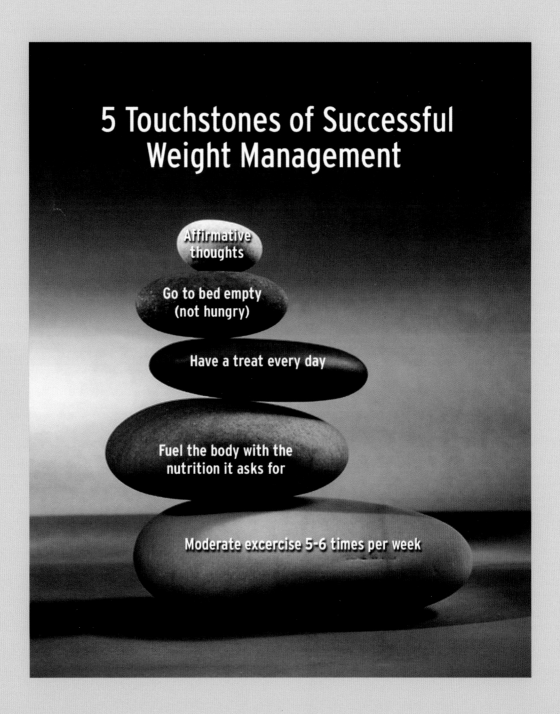

5 Touchstones of Successful Weight Management

Affirmative thoughts

Go to bed empty (not hungry)

Have a treat every day

Fuel the body with the nutrition it asks for

Moderate excercise 5-6 times per week

Reasons to Exercise

Do you need a reason to exercise? Here are a few key benefits of exercising today:

- Keeps the body moving—because if you don't use it, you lose it!

- Speeds up the metabolism.

- Burns fat.

- Oxygenates body & brain.

- Improves cognitive functions—studies show exercise makes you smarter.

Remove this page and post it where you will see it daily.